REVISION GUIDE

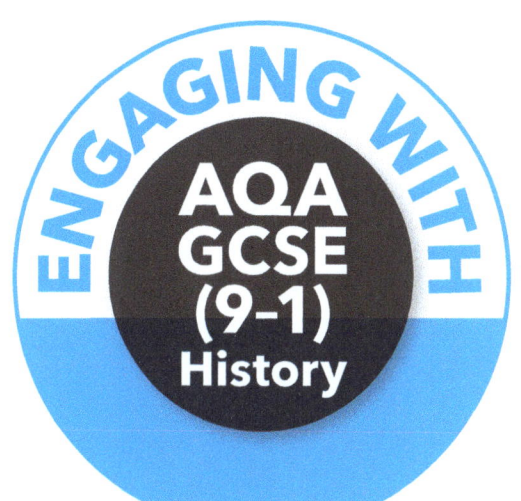

HEALTH & THE PEOPLE c1000 TO THE PRESENT DAY

THEMATIC STUDY

DALE BANHAM

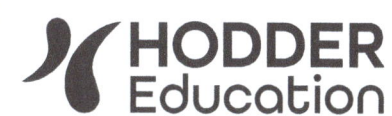

The Publishers would like to thank the following for permission to reproduce copyright material.

Photo credits

p.24 & 32 Wellcome Collection, London/http://creativecommons.org/licenses/by/4.0/

Acknowledgements

Every effort has been made to trace all copyright holders, but if any have been inadvertently overlooked, the Publishers will be pleased to make the necessary arrangements at the first opportunity.

Although every effort has been made to ensure that website addresses are correct at time of going to press, Hodder Education cannot be held responsible for the content of any website mentioned in this book. It is sometimes possible to find a relocated web page by typing in the address of the home page for a website in the URL window of your browser.

Hachette UK's policy is to use papers that are natural, renewable and recyclable products and made from wood grown in well-managed forests and other controlled sources. The logging and manufacturing processes are expected to conform to the environmental regulations of the country of origin.

Orders: please contact Hachette UK Distribution, Hely Hutchinson Centre, Milton Road, Didcot, Oxfordshire, OX11 7HH. Telephone: +44 (0)1235 827827. Email education@hachette.co.uk Lines are open from 9 a.m. to 5 p.m., Monday to Friday. You can also order through our website: www.hoddereducation.co.uk

ISBN: 978 1 3983 8523 8

© Dale Banham 2023

First published in 2023 by
Hodder Education,
An Hachette UK Company
Carmelite House
50 Victoria Embankment
London EC4Y 0DZ

www.hoddereducation.co.uk

Impression number 10 9 8 7 6 5 4 3 2 1

Year   2027 2026 2025 2024 2023

All rights reserved. Apart from any use permitted under UK copyright law, no part of this publication may be reproduced or transmitted in any form or by any means, electronic or mechanical, including photocopying and recording, or held within any information storage and retrieval system, without permission in writing from the publisher or under licence from the Copyright Licensing Agency Limited. Further details of such licences (for reprographic reproduction) may be obtained from the Copyright Licensing Agency Limited, www.cla.co.uk

Cover photo: 'An ill man who is being bled by his doctor. Coloured etching by J. Sneyd, 1804, after J. Gillray.' by James Gillray. Wellcome Collection. CC BY

Illustrations by Aptara, Inc.

Typeset in India by Aptara, Inc.

Printed in the UK at Ashford Colour Press LTD

A catalogue record for this title is available from the British Library.

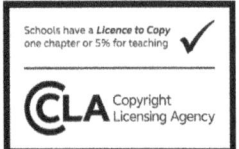

CONTENTS

Introduction: How to prepare for the exam   4

Part 1: The Middle Ages, c1000–1500: Medicine stands still

- **Knowledge tests:** How much do you know about medicine in the Middle Ages?   6
- **Core content 1.1:** Medieval medicine   8
- **Core content 1.2:** Medical progress in the Middle Ages   10
- **Core content 1.3:** Public health in the Middle Ages   12
- **Apply:** Exam practice   14

Part 2: Renaissance Britain, c1500–1800: The beginnings of change

- **Knowledge tests:** How much do you know about medicine in Renaissance Britain?   16
- **Core content 2.1:** The impact of the Renaissance on Britain   18
- **Core content 2.2:** Dealing with disease   20
- **Core content 2.3:** Prevention of disease   22
- **Apply:** Exam practice   23

Part 3: The nineteenth century, c1800–1900: A revolution in medicine

- **Knowledge tests:** How much do you know about medicine in the nineteenth century?   26
- **Core content 3.1:** The development of the Germ Theory and its impact on the treatment of disease in Britain   28
- **Core content 3.2:** A revolution in surgery   30
- **Core content 3.3:** Improvements in public health   32
- **Apply:** Exam practice   34

Part 4: Modern medicine, c1900–today

- **Knowledge tests:** How much do you know about modern medicine?   36
- **Core content 4.1:** Modern treatment of disease   38
- **Core content 4.2:** The impact of war and technology on surgery   40
- **Core content 4.3:** Modern public health   42
- **Apply:** Exam practice   44

The Big Picture of medicine and health, c1000–the present day   46

Glossary   48

How this book helps you revise and improve your grades

As you can see from this contents page, the book matches the exam specification and is divided into four time periods. You have already covered these with your teacher so each chapter starts with a set of **knowledge tests** so that you can find out how much can you remember about each time period and plan a revision programme where you close gaps in your knowledge.

The **core content** pages will provide the answers to the questions you struggled with. These are designed in the style of flashcards so that you don't have to make your own and you can spend more time re-testing yourself and practising exam questions.

The book also shows you how to apply your knowledge to answer exam questions. Just knowing lots of information is not enough. The **Apply: Exam practice** pages at the end of each chapter will show you what to do with that knowledge so that you gain a high grade.

Introduction: How to prepare for the exam

Your exam: What is assessed and how

Your AQA GCSE (9–1) History course is made up of four different studies. These are assessed in two exam papers.

Paper 1: Understanding the modern world (2 hours)	Paper 2: Shaping the nation (2 hours)
Section A: Period study This focuses on key developments in a country's history over at least a 50-year period.	**Section A: Thematic Study** This looks at key developments in Britain over a long period of time (at least 800 years).
Section B: Wider world depth study This focuses on international conflict and tension over a period of 20–25 years.	**Section B: British depth study** This focuses on a period of British history over a short period of time (under 40 years).

This book prepares you for Section A of Paper 2 – **Britain: Health and the People: c1000 to the present day**. The table below shows you how the Thematic Study will be examined.

	Type of question	Guidance	Marks	Timing	Advice and practice
1	How useful is Source …	The source could be visual or written. It will relate to a key event, development or individual. Focus on **why** the source is useful. Use the content of the source, the provenance (Who produced it? When? Why?) and your contextual knowledge (What was happening at the time?) to evaluate the usefulness of the source.	8	10 minutes	Pages 23 and 34
2	Explain the significance of …	Think then **and** now. What was the importance of a key event, individual or development at the time (short-term impact)? AND … What was the importance over time (long-term consequences, influence today)?	8	10 minutes	Pages 24 and 35
3	Compare … In what ways are they similar/ different?	Focus on the question – focus on similarities **or** differences; you do not need to do both. Identify and explain ways in which the two events are similar/different. Think: • Are the reasons why the two events happened similar/different? • Are there similarities/differences in how the event developed or how people responded? • Are there similarities/differences in the impacts, outcomes or results of the event?	8	10 minutes	Pages 25 and 35
4	Evaluate factors	This is an essay question, requiring you to reach a **judgement**. Aim to evaluate the factor stated in the question first. Weigh how important it was compared to **two** other factors. Reach a judgement – was it the most important factor? Use your knowledge of all four parts of the specification to support your argument.	20 (16 + 4 for SPaG)	25 minutes	Pages 14, 33, 35 and 44

Your exam: The key steps to success

This book uses the latest research into effective revision strategies to help you remember the core content. The specification is divided into 4 time periods so follow the structure of the book and break your revision down into 4 parts. For each time period, follow the steps below. They will help you revise more effectively – saving you time and boosting your grade.

Step 1: Test your knowledge of a time period
Start by using the **knowledge tests** at the start of each chapter. Testing yourself is a great way to start your revision as it boosts memory.

When you test yourself, your memory of that information gets significantly stronger. Our brains are also hard-wired to learn from our mistakes. You will be able to check your answers to the knowledge tests using the page numbers provided.

Step 2: Identify gaps in your knowledge
Use the knowledge tests to show you where you need to focus your revision.

Your time is precious, so you need to make sure that you focus on revising your weaker topics. Too many students spend too much time revising topics they already know very well!

Step 3: Use the core content pages to close the gaps in your knowledge
The core content pages in this book will help you improve your knowledge and understanding of your weaker topics. At the top of these pages, a **checklist of the core content** from the specification is provided so that you can identify topics that you need to focus on.

At key points, **memory aids** are provided to help you remember key individuals or developments in medicine and health. They use images or diagrams but very few words. Most people remember better if something is summarised with both text and images.

Step 4: Apply your knowledge and understanding to exam questions
When you feel confident with the content for each time period, use the **Apply: Exam practice** pages in the book to gain a strong understanding of how to approach each of the four exam questions (see page 4). Our practice questions are like the questions you will be asked in the exam. You can get past papers from your teacher or from the AQA website.

We provide **Exam Tips** for each question type – showing you how to approach it and improve your grades.

Step 5: Review your exam answers and respond to feedback
This book provides model answers that highlight the key features of high-quality written work. The **Apply: Exam practice** pages also provide **Exam Tips** that you can use to review your own work. Use the advice provided as a checklist to reflect on your own answers.

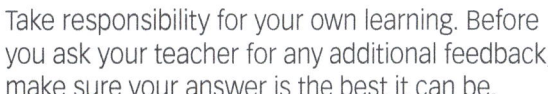

Take responsibility for your own learning. Before you ask your teacher for any additional feedback, make sure your answer is the best it can be.

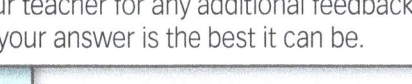

Part 1 The Middle Ages, c1000–1500: Medicine stands still

🚦 Knowledge tests: How much do you know about medicine in the Middle Ages?

It may seem strange starting your revision with a knowledge test but remember this is the best way to boost your memory and it will help you identify gaps in your knowledge. Do not worry if you cannot answer all the questions or if you make mistakes. You can use the **Core content** pages to check your answers and fill in the gaps in your knowledge.

> **Revision Tip**
>
> When you have finished all the **Recall challenges**, use the page references in blue to check your answers. If you have made a mistake, use a different colour pen to write in the correct answer.

Recall challenges ▶

1: Know the key individuals

Knowing the main individuals that influenced medicine in each time period will really help you in the exam. Think of each individual as a hook on which you can hang other knowledge.

Task
Match each individual with the correct description.

Key individual	How their work influenced the development of medicine
Hippocrates	• An Islamic doctor who wrote *The Canon of Medicine*. • This became the main medical textbook for physicians until the seventeenth century (1600s). It described over 700 drugs and medicines and their uses, and how to diagnose illness.
Galen	• A Greek doctor who taught that people got ill because their humours were out of balance. • He taught doctors to examine patients carefully and to observe their symptoms. His ideas influenced Galen.
Ibn Sina (or Avicenna)	• A British surgeon who worked for the King. He designed a new forcep that could remove an arrowhead. • He also used barley and honey to help wounds heal free from any infection.
Al-Razi (or Rhazes)	• A French surgeon who was influenced by the work of Galen and Islamic doctors such as Ibn Sina and Al-Razi. • He wrote a book on surgery that was widely used in England in the Middle Ages. It covered bloodletting, the use of bandages, cauterisation and how to treat wounds and fractures.
John Bradmore	• An Islamic doctor who wrote over 50 books based on the ideas of Hippocrates and Galen, as well as ideas from China and India. • His books were widely used in Europe in the Middle Ages – they stressed that it was important for physicians to carefully diagnose illness before deciding on a treatment.
Guy de Chauliac	• A Roman doctor who wrote more than 350 books which were used to train doctors in the Middle Ages. • He developed the Theory of Opposites to balance the humours and produced detailed description of the human anatomy.

2: Know the key terms

As you revise, it is important to check your understanding of subject-specific vocabulary. The topic you are studying contains some important key terms.

Task
Match each key term with its correct definition or description.

Key term	Definition
Superstition	The idea of using 'opposites' to balance the humours. For example, if a patient had too much phlegm, caused by cold, they would be given hot food such as peppers.
The Theory of the Four Humours	A plague that killed over 40 per cent of the population of England during the Middle Ages.
The Theory of Opposites	A building where monks lived and devoted their time to worshiping God.
Bloodletting	The understanding of the structure and make-up of the body.
The Black Death	The belief that people became ill because liquids in the body were out of balance.
Cauterisation	Using a hot iron to burn body tissue. This seals a wound and stops it bleeding.
Anatomy	The treatment of opening a vein or applying leeches to draw blood from a patient.
Physician	An unscientific belief based on ignorance or fear. For example, a belief based on supernatural influences, or good or bad luck.
Monasteries	The highest-ranking doctors. They were well paid and tended to treat the rich people in England.

3: The ten-minute quiz

Test your ability to remember information under pressure. The more you do this, the more you will be prepared for the time pressures of the exam.

Task
- Answer as many of the questions below as you can in ten minutes.
- Mark your work, using the page numbers provided. A total of 50 marks are available.
- Use the quiz to identify areas you need to revise in detail. If you have made a mistake, **use a different colour pen to write in the correct answer**. This will help you to identify gaps in your knowledge and decide the topics you need to focus on to improve your knowledge and understanding.

List three things that people believed caused illness.	List three key features of **Galenic medicine** (based on the ideas of Galen).	List the **four humours**.	See pages 8–9 for the answers.	Mark out of 10
List three common treatments for illness.	List three types of people who treated the sick.	List two methods of diagnosing illness.		Mark out of 8
List three ways that Christianity had a positive impact on medicine and health care.	List two ways that Christianity provided an obstacle to medical progress.	List three ways that doctors in England were influenced by the work of Islamic doctors.	See pages 10–11 for the answers.	Mark out of 8
List three treatments offered by barber-surgeons.	List three problems faced by surgeons in the Middle Ages.	List two surgeons who introduced new surgical methods.		Mark out of 8
List three public health problems that existed in medieval towns.	List three public health improvements that took place in towns.	List two positive features of public health in monasteries.	See pages 12–13 for the answers.	Mark out of 8
List three ways that people tried to prevent the spread of the Black Death.	List three treatments for the Black Death.	List two consequences of the Black Death.		Mark out of 8

Core content 1.1: Medieval medicine

Exam specification checklist for this topic

- Beliefs about the cause of illness
- Methods used to diagnose and treat illness
- The key features of Hippocratic and Galenic medicine
- Medieval doctors and how they were trained

Revision task

Use the flashcards on pages 8–9 to improve your knowledge and understanding of these topics. Test yourself by trying to answer the key questions with the bullet point answers covered up. Make a note of the topics you struggle to remember – you can spend more time on them later in your revision programme.

Key question 1: What did people believe caused illness and disease in the Middle Ages?

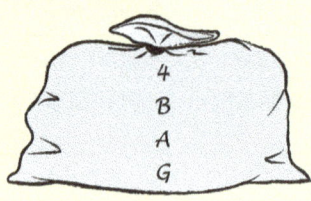

- **Four humours** – People got ill when one of the four humours in their body was out of balance. Doctors would test a patient's urine to judge if a patient's humours were in balance.
- **Bad air** caused illness – Some people linked bad air to filthy streets (but they could not explain the link).
- **Astrology** – Doctors believed that the movement of the sun and the planets affected people's bodies. They used a zodiac chart to work out when to treat each part of the body.
- **God** – Most people believed that illness was sent by God, as a punishment for their sins.

Key question 2: What was the Theory of the Four Humours?

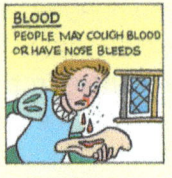 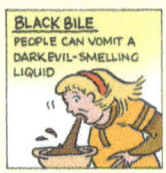
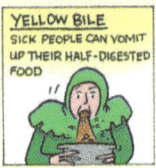 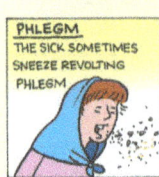

- This was a theory developed by a doctor from Ancient Greece called Hippocrates.
- He said that the body was made up of four humours (or liquids) and that when people became ill these humours were out of balance. He said that when people were sick, they needed to get rid of the humour that they had too much of.
- A famous Roman doctor called Galen built on Hippocrates' ideas (see below).

Key question 3: What were the key features of Galenic medicine?

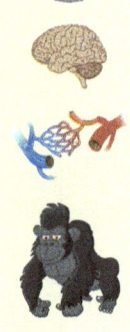

- Galen said that doctors should **balance** the four humours, using the Theory of Opposites. For example, if a patient had too much phlegm, then the illness was caused by cold. Galen's treatment was the opposite – he gave the patient hot food, such as peppers.
- Galen carried out experiments on animals such as pigs to prove that the **brain** controlled speech.
- Galen proved that **blood** was carried around the body by the arteries and the veins.
- Galen carried out dissections to try to find out about anatomy (the structure of the **body**). When he could not use human bodies, he used apes. This led to some mistakes. For example, the human jaw bone is made from one bone, not two (as in apes).
- Galen wrote over 350 **books** which covered every aspect of medicine. People believed his books contained all the answers and they were used to train doctors for the next 1500 years. Galen taught that the body had been created by one God and this fitted in with the ideas of the Christian Church. As a result, few people challenged his ideas.

Key question 4: How was illness treated in the Middle Ages?

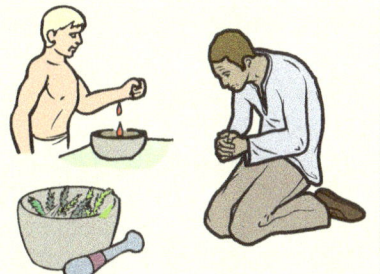

- **Bleeding** – People were bled regularly to avoid illness. A surgeon or doctor would balance a patient's humours by letting blood flow from the arm. They sometimes used leeches to suck out the blood.
- **Herbal remedies** – The most common treatments were made from herbs, minerals and animal parts. Some potions/treatments were based on superstition, but others worked. For example, many included honey which is known to fight infection.
- **Prayer** – As illness was seen as a punishment from God, people would pray for members of their family to become better or say prayers while collecting herbs (in order to increase the effectiveness of the treatment).

Key question 5: Who treated the sick?	**Physicians** – the highest-ranking doctors	**Women** or a **local wise woman**	**Surgeons**
Who did they treat?	Rich people – in 1300, there were fewer than 100 physicians in England	Family members, people in their local village	People with a small amount of money
How did they diagnose illness?	• Zodiac chart • Urine chart (showing if the colour, thickness or smell of the urine meant the humours were out of balance)	• Observation and using previous experiences	• Some read books by European or Arab surgeons
How did they treat illness?	• Bleeding • Purging (making a patient vomit) • Encouraging exercise and regular washing	• Herbal remedies	• Bleeding • Amputations
How were they trained?	• University • Read Galen's books • Watched dissections (designed to show that Galen was correct!)	• Knowledge passed on by their mother or grandmother	• Apprentices to experienced surgeons

Core content 1.2: Medical progress in the Middle Ages

Exam specification checklist for this topic
- The contribution of Christianity to medical progress and treatment
- Hospitals in the Middle Ages
- The importance of Islamic medicine and surgery
- Surgery in the Middle Ages

Revision task
Use the flashcards on pages 10–11 to improve your knowledge and understanding of these topics. Test yourself by trying to answer the key questions with the bullet point answers covered up. Make a note of the topics you struggle to remember – you can spend more time on them later in your revision programme.

Key question 1: How far did Christianity help medicine progress during the Middle Ages?	The Christian Church had a big influence on everyone's ideas in the Middle Ages. Ideas spread from the Pope in Rome, through the archbishops and bishops, to the priest in every village in Britain.

Area of medicine	The influence of Christianity
Preserving knowledge	The Christian Church helped to preserve knowledge. Monks made copies of books so that doctors in the Middle Ages could learn from the ideas of people like Galen.
Knowledge about the cause of disease	The Church said that God controlled all aspects of life, so people believed that God caused illness. This meant that they did not look for other causes.
Treatments	If illness was a punishment for sin, then there was also no need to develop new treatments. You just had to be more religious, pray more and commit fewer sins.
Education and training	The Church controlled the universities where physicians trained. The Church liked Galen's ideas because his books supported the Christian belief that God created human beings. Physicians were encouraged to accept Galen's ideas; they were punished if they challenged them or started to do their own research.
Care for the sick	The Christian Church taught that sick people should be looked after. This led to many hospitals being set up (see Key question 2 below).

Key question 2: What were the key features of hospitals in the Middle Ages?	**Organisation** – Who set up and ran the hospitals?	The Christian Church – hospitals were set up in monasteries
	Staffing – Who provided the medical care?	Not physicians Mainly nuns
	Patients – Who did they treat?	Rarely the sick Mainly the poor and the elderly
	Treatments – How were these patients treated?	Mainly prayer, rest and food Some herbal remedies
	Scale – How many hospitals were there?	500 (by 1400) But mainly small, with about ten patients in each

Key question 3: How did Islamic doctors and surgeons influence the development of medicine and surgery in Britain?	• Islamic doctors helped to preserve the ideas of the Ancient Greeks and Romans. They wrote medical encyclopaedias which carefully organised medical knowledge so the work of people from the past, like Galen, could be studied by European physicians. • Islamic doctors also added their own research. The work of key individuals was translated into Latin and used in medical schools in England to train physicians. • **Al-Razi** (or Rhazes) wrote over 50 books based on the ideas of Hippocrates and Galen, as well as Chinese and Indian sources. His books were used for centuries after his death in AD925. They emphasised the importance of the physician carefully diagnosing the illness. • **Al-Zahrawi** (or Albucasis) produced a 30-volume encyclopaedia of medical practices. The chapter on surgery was translated into Latin and became widely used in Europe. His work included illustrations of more than 200 surgical instruments. • **Ibn Sina** (or Avicenna) wrote *The Canon of Medicine* – this became the main medical textbook for physicians in Europe during the Middle Ages. It described over 700 drugs and medicines and their uses, and how to diagnose diseases.
Key question 4: Who were barber-surgeons and how did they treat people?	• Most surgery in the Middle Ages was performed by barber-surgeons. They offered blood-letting, tooth extractions and amputations, as well as haircuts and shaves! • They could also remove small tumours on the skin's surface. • However, they could not do complex operations inside the body.
Key question 5: Why did surgeons in the Middle Ages face a PILE of problems? 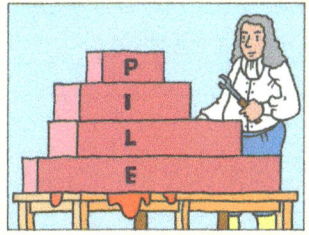	• **Pain** – Some surgeons used herbs such as opium or hemlock to make patients drowsy, but these could kill the patient if too big a dose was used. There was no effective way to relieve pain during an operation. • **Infections** – Wine, vinegar or honey were used to clean wounds, but these did not prevent infections spreading. • **Loss of blood** – Large cuts were sewn up and often cauterised to prevent loss of blood (this involved closing wounds by sealing them with a burning iron). • **Environment** – Surgeons did not have clean rooms to operate in and germs could easily be spread in this kind of environment. Surgeons did not wear masks, gowns or gloves.
Key question 6: What new methods were introduced by surgeons in the Middle Ages? 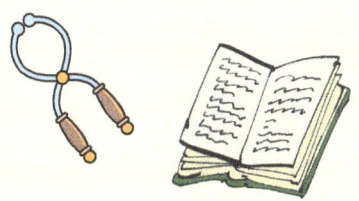	**John Bradmore** was a royal surgeon who designed a new forcep to remove an arrowhead. He did this to save the life of Henry, Prince of Wales, wounded during a battle after an arrow had passed through his cheek and lodged in the bottom of his skull. **Guy de Chauliac** was a French surgeon whose book told surgeons how to carry out bloodletting and cauterisation, as well as how to treat cataracts, hernias and bone fractures. He was heavily influenced by the work of Islamic doctors such as Ibn Sina.

Core content 1.3: Public health in the Middle Ages

Exam specification checklist for this topic
- Public health conditions in medieval towns
- Public health conditions in medieval monasteries

Revision task
Use the flashcards on pages 12–13 to improve your knowledge and understanding of these topics. Test yourself by trying to answer the key questions with the bullet point answers covered up. Make a note of the topics you struggle to remember – you can spend more time on them later in your revision programme.

Key question 1: What public health problems existed in medieval towns?

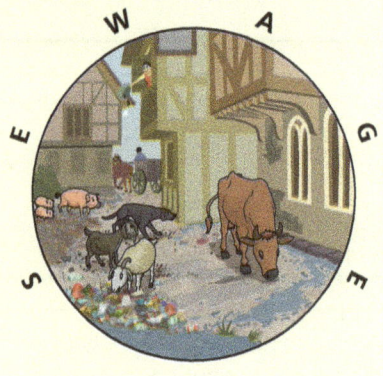

- **Sewers** – There were no underground sewers. Open sewers or drains ran through the streets.
- **Environment** – The whole environment was very unclean. Rubbish and human excrement were thrown into the streets. Towns could be very overcrowded, and houses were built close together. This meant that disease spread quickly.
- **Water** – There was a lack of clean drinking water. Cesspits for human waste were sometimes built near water supplies (such as wells). People threw rubbish (including human excrement) into the rivers that were used as a water supply.
- **Animals** – Cattle, sheep and pigs roamed the streets. Horses were used for transport. These animals left dung. Butchers threw animal remains into the streets.
- **Government** – The government did introduce some measures to try to improve public health (see below) but it was not enough to deal with the scale of the problem. Laws were not fully enforced, and not enough people were employed to keep the streets clean.
- **Epidemics** – Diseases such as plague were common and epidemics (diseases that spread very quickly) killed many people.

Key question 2: What public health improvements were introduced in towns?

- In Exeter, **aqueducts** were built to bring fresh water into the town.
- Rakers were employed to clean the streets and remove animal dung.
- Night **carts** collected human waste from cesspits.
- **Cesspits** were lined with brick or stone so they did not leak into water supplies.
- **Laws** were passed to punish people for throwing human or butchers' waste into the streets.

Key question 3: What were the key features of public health in monasteries?

- The best public health facilities were in monasteries. Monasteries were wealthy. This was because rich people gave them money in return for prayers. This allowed monasteries to install water supplies and latrines (toilets).
- Monks were expected to keep clean. They washed their clothes regularly. Monasteries were often close to rivers and built away from town centres. This gave the monks a fresh water supply.

Key question 4: What caused the Black Death?	The Black Death spread across Europe after arriving from Asia, reaching England in 1348. It was a combination of two diseases.
	• The main disease was **bubonic plague** – carried by rats and spread by fleas. Victims felt cold and tired, then got painful swellings called buboes (as big as eggs) on their neck and in their groin or armpits. These were quickly followed by high fever, severe headache, then usually death after three days.
	• The epidemic was made worse by **pneumonic plague** – spread by people coughing over others. Victims coughed up blood and died within a day or two from this plague.

Key question 5: How did people try to prevent the Black Death from spreading?	• Kind Edward III wrote to the Mayor of London, ordering him to clean the streets. He said that 'bad odours' from rubbish were causing the disease to spread.
	• Bishops ordered daily processions and church services to ask for God's help.
	• People carried sweet-smelling herbs or lit fires to overpower the bad air.
	• People fasted (stopped eating) to show they were sorry for their sins.
	• People punished themselves in public and begged for God's forgiveness. For example, flagellants walked through the streets of London, whipping themselves to show God that they repented their sins.
	• Doors and windows were shut and sealed.

Key question 6: How did people try to treat the Black Death?

Complete the table below to show the links between the methods of treatment and beliefs about the cause.

Method of treatment	The belief about cause
Prayers for sufferers to recover	God
Holy charms around the necks of the sick	
Leeches to bleed patients	
Treatment by opposites – as patients had a fever, cold baths were used	

Key question 7: What were the consequences of the Black Death?	**Short-term consequences:**
	• The Black Death killed over one-third of the population in 12 months. It affected both rich and poor.
	• Towns and ports were the hardest hit. Only remote villages and farms avoided it.
	Long-term consequences:
	• The death of so many workers led to food shortages and food prices increased.
	• However, over time, survivors became better off. There was a shortage of workers, so employers had to pay higher wages to attract them.
	• As a result, people had more money to spend on education. More people learned to read and write, which helped spread new ideas more quickly.

Apply: Exam practice

Question 4: How to evaluate the key factors

Question 4 in the exam is worth 16 marks – nearly half the marks for the 'Health and the People' exam paper. This question will test your knowledge and understanding of the key factors that have influenced how medicine developed in each time period. The focus here is on causation – you will need to explain why medicine developed in the way that it did.

> **Revision Tip**
>
> The key factors identified in the exam specification are shown in the table below. The third column shows how each factor played a role in the development of medicine in the Middle Ages.
>
> Remember to produce factors tables for the other three time periods. Use them regularly as part of your revision programme. Cover up the information in the right-hand column and see if you can recall an example of the role played by each of the factors.

Factors	Explanation	Example(s) from the Middle Ages
Beliefs	Religious beliefs have both encouraged and inhibited change.	• The Church set up hospitals and encouraged care for the sick. • Monks preserved and spread knowledge by making copies of ancient medical books. • The Church set up universities where physicians were trained. • The Church discouraged people from challenging Galen and developing new ideas.
Individuals	Individuals have influenced medicine by developing new ideas or inventions.	• Doctors in Britain were influenced by the work of Islamic doctors such as Al-Razi, Al-Zahrawi and Ibn Sina.
Government	Governments can pass laws to improve public health and they can fund new developments and health care.	• During the Black Death, Edward III ordered that the streets in London should be cleaned.
Communication	Medical books have helped to preserve knowledge from the past and spread new ideas.	• People in Britain were influenced by books written by Galen. • Surgeons were influenced by books written by Guy de Chauliac.
Chance	Sometimes, new discoveries are made by chance.	• See below (John Bradmore)
War	New surgical techniques can be developed during wartime because there are so many serious injuries to treat.	• Bradmore developed a new forcep to remove arrowheads when Prince Henry was injured on the battlefield.
Science and technology	Developments in science and technology can lead to new inventions that change the way illness is diagnosed, prevented and treated.	• This factor has tended to have its biggest impact in the last 200 years.

Communicating your knowledge and understanding about causation

For Question 4 you need to explain the role played by factors in the development of medicine.

Look at the example paragraph below – it argues that the causal factor of communication played an important role in the development of surgery during the Middle Ages. When arguing the importance of a factor, you cannot simply *say* that it was important. You have to *prove* it was. The paragraph below has two important features that will help you move your answer into the higher levels of the mark scheme.

Feature 1

It is a **developed** answer. Phrases like 'this meant that', 'this led to' and 'this resulted in' are called causal connectives because they tie what you know to the question and help you prove your argument.

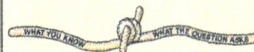

Communication was an important factor that helped medicine progress during the medieval period. Books were produced by Islamic doctors that preserved knowledge from the Ancient Greeks and included new ideas about the way the body worked. **This meant that** doctors in Britain and other parts of Europe could learn ideas from other cultures. **For example**, Avicenna's medical encyclopaedia, 'The Canon of Medicine', was used to teach European physicians until the 1600s. In addition, surgeons in Britain had access to carefully illustrated books on surgical techniques. **This led to** the spread of surgical techniques and old ideas, **such as** the belief that pus helped wounds heal, being challenged. Guy de Chauliac wrote a seven-volume book on surgery and this demonstrates the detailed knowledge that medieval surgeons could draw on to develop their surgical skills.

Feature 2

It is a **substantiated** answer – this means that the answer is supported by specific examples. Use phrases like 'for example' and 'such as' to introduce your supporting evidence.

Use the sentence starters below to write a paragraph on the role played by religious beliefs in the development of medicine in the Middle Ages. Remember to include causal connectives to develop your explanation and provide specific examples to support the points you make.

Religion played an important role in influencing medicine and public health in the medieval period. Epidemics **such as** … were seen as a punishment from God. **This meant that** people did not look for scientific explanations of disease and did not make the link between illness and poor public health facilities.

Galen's ideas fitted in well with Christianity. **This led to** …

However, the influence of religion also improved some areas of medicine. **For example**, …

Revision Tip

Keep revisiting the memory aids

The memory aids we have provided help you remember the key points about the main areas of medicine. Use the memory aids below to answer these questions about the Middle Ages.

- What did people believe caused illness and disease?

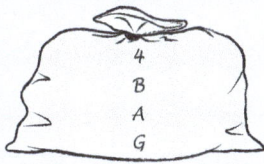

page 8

- Why did surgeons face problems?

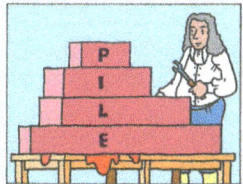

page 11

- What public health problems existed in towns?

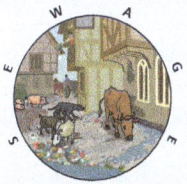

page 12

Part 2 Renaissance Britain, c1500–1800: The beginnings of change

Knowledge tests: How much do you know about medicine in Renaissance Britain?

Recall challenges

1: Know the key individuals

Task

Match each of the individuals in the box below with the area of medicine that they helped to develop.

Individual	What areas of medicine did they influence?
Andreas Vesalius	**Surgery and medical training** (he even trained Jenner)
William Harvey	**Prevention** of disease – developed the first vaccination
Ambroise Paré	**Surgery** – introduced new methods to help injured soldiers
Joshua Ward	**Anatomy** – published *The Fabrica* – a book detailing the structure of the human body
John Hunter	**Treatment** – but not in a good way – his 'cure-all' pill just made people sweat a lot
James Morrison	**Treatment** – but definitely not in a good way – his 'Vegetable Pills' caused deaths due to excessive bowel movements!
Edward Jenner	**Physiology** – improved knowledge about the way the body worked (in this case the heart)

2: The ten-minute quiz

List two of Galen's theories about anatomy that Vesalius proved wrong.	List three ways in which Vesalius was significant.	List three new surgical methods introduced by Paré.	See pages 18–19 for the answers.	Mark out of 8
List two key theories about physiology developed by Harvey.	List three ways in which Harvey influenced medicine in the longer term.	List three ways in which Hunter was significant.		Mark out of 8
List two common treatments for illness that continued from the Middle Ages.	List three new treatments introduced from abroad.	List two types of pills, sold by quacks, that did not help people at the time.	See pages 20–21 for the answers.	Mark out of 7
List three ways that the Mayor of London tried to prevent the spread of the plague.	List two ways that hospitals changed in the eighteenth century.	List two ways in which the training of doctors improved.		Mark out of 7

How did people try to prevent smallpox before Jenner?	What mild disease prevented people from getting smallpox?	Why did it take so long for another vaccination to be developed?	See pages 22–23 for the answers.	Mark out of 3
List three reasons why Jenner faced opposition.	List two ways in which the government played an important role in the fight against smallpox.	List two ways in which Jenner tried to prove that his smallpox vaccine worked.		Mark out of 7

Task

1. Using the table below, cover up the second column and see how much you can remember about health and the people in the Middle Ages. Highlight key points you missed.
2. Now add in information you can remember about the Renaissance period. You can check your answer using the period summary of the Renaissance on page 49 of the student book. Add in things you missed in a different colour. You can use the **Core content** pages in this chapter to learn about these developments and close the gaps in your knowledge and understanding.

Theme	The Middle Ages, c1000–1500	Renaissance Britain, c1500–1800
Ideas about the causes of illness	• Four humours • Bad air (miasma) • Astrology – movement of the planets • God – a punishment for sins	
Knowledge of the human body (anatomy)	• Doctors followed ideas of Galen and knew about Greek, Roman and Arab discoveries • Doctors encouraged to accept traditional ideas – not make new discoveries • Dissections were done to illustrate what Galen had said	
Treatments	• Prayers and charms • Remedies using herbs, minerals and animal parts • Bleeding and purging to restore the balance of the humours (Galen's Theory of Opposites) • Rest, exercise and diet	
Surgery	• Simple surgery on visible tumours and wounds; splints for fractured bones • Plants such as opium dulled pain but there were no effective anaesthetics • Wine, vinegar or honey used to clean wounds but could not prevent infections • Large wounds stitched or cauterisation used to stop heavy bleeding	
Public health and methods of prevention	• Kings and governments not expected to improve public health • Epidemic diseases and plagues could not be stopped • Towns employed rakers and made laws but struggled to keep streets clean • Animal and human waste in streets; open sewers; lack of clean water	
Hospitals and healers	• Mothers and family members treated most illnesses • Physicians trained at university but only treated the rich • Hospitals set up by the Church but were very small • Care provided by nuns; mainly offered rest, food and prayers	

Core content 2.1: The impact of the Renaissance on Britain

Exam specification checklist for this topic

- How Vesalius challenged traditional ideas about anatomy
- How Harvey challenged traditional ideas about physiology
- How Paré developed new methods in surgery
- How Hunter developed the study of anatomy and surgery
- Why there was opposition to change?

Revision task

Use the flashcards on pages 18–19 to improve your knowledge and understanding of these topics. Test yourself by trying to answer the key questions with the bullet point answers covered up. Make a note of the topics you struggle to remember – you can spend more time on them later in your revision programme.

Key question 1: Why was the work of Vesalius significant?

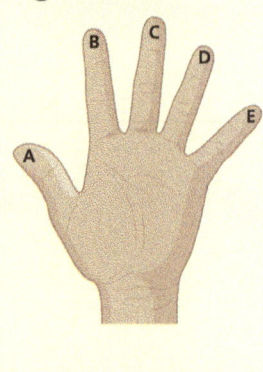

- **Anatomy** – Andreas Vesalius was a Belgian doctor, born in 1514, who helped to improve knowledge about anatomy.
- **Book** – Vesalius published *The Fabric of the Human Body*. This book was full of illustrations that showed the body in far more detail than ever before. The invention of the printing press meant that the book was widely available to doctors all over Europe. By the 1560s, it was being used in Britain to train doctors.
- **Challenged** – Vesalius challenged traditional ideas. He proved that Galen made some mistakes. For example, the human jaw bone is made from one bone, not two (as Galen had said).
- **Dissection** – Vesalius encouraged doctors to carry out their own dissections.
- **Education** – At first, many doctors stuck to traditional ideas, thinking it was wrong to challenge Galen. However, in the longer term, the education and training of doctors began to change. By the late 1600s, most students were encouraged to find things out for themselves and gain hands-on experience through dissections.

Key question 2: Why was the work of Harvey significant?

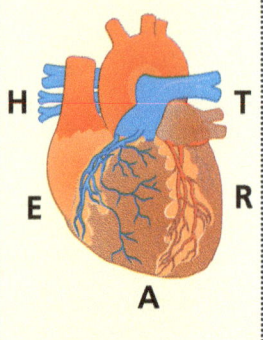

- **Heart** – William Harvey was an English doctor, born in 1578, who proved that the heart pumped blood around the body. His theory of the way that blood circulated around the body challenged Galen, who had taught that the liver produced blood and it was burnt up in the body.
- **Experiments** – Through experiments, Harvey developed new ideas about physiology (the way the body works) and was able to prove his ideas. He encouraged other doctors to carry out their own research.
- **Arteries** – Harvey showed how the body has a one-way system for the blood. Arteries carry blood away from the heart. Harvey used finger pressure demonstrations to show that valves in veins direct blood towards the heart.
- **Royal Society** – Harvey's work inspired others and, in 1660, the Royal Society was established. Members met weekly to discuss ideas and carry out experiments. The Society published books to spread new ideas.
- **Turning point** – At first, many doctors ignored Harvey's ideas. However, in the longer term, Harvey's ideas were accepted by universities. This was an important turning point as many areas of medicine have been influenced by Harvey's work. For example:
  - heart surgery – depends on a precise understanding of how the heart works
  - injections – depend on knowing how blood circulates
  - Harvey's theories explained how poisons could spread so quickly through the body.

Key question 3: Why was there opposition to the ideas of Vesalius and Harvey?	• The ideas of important individuals such as Vesalius and Harvey were slow to catch on. Many doctors said it was wrong to challenge Galen. Their **medical training** taught that Galen had given a fully correct description of anatomy so there was no point trying to find things out for themselves. • The work of Vesalius and Harvey **did not have an immediate impact** on understanding disease or treatments. In the short term, no one was healthier as a result of Vesalius' or Harvey's work.
Key question 4: How did Paré change surgery? 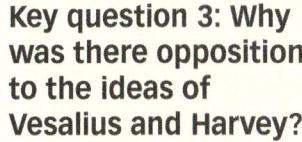	• **Limbs** (artificial) – Ambroise Paré was a French surgeon, born in 1510, who designed false limbs for wounded soldiers. In total, he designed more than 50 false body parts and included drawings of them in his books to spread the idea. Skilled armourers made the false limbs – the mechanisms inside the false hands they made were so good they allowed a soldier to hold a sword and fight. • **Lotions** – Before Paré, surgeons thought that the only way to stop wounds becoming poisoned by gunpowder was to pour boiling oil over them. However, on one occasion on the battlefield, Paré ran out of oil. Instead, he mixed up an ointment (lotion) made from egg yolks, turpentine and oil of roses. He found that this new method reduced pain and stopped wounds from becoming infected. Through his books, Paré's method of treating gunshot wounds became widely accepted in Britain. • **Ligatures** – Paré saw how cauterising wounds (using a hot iron to burn body tissue and seal a wound) caused patients extreme pain and did not always stop bleeding. He experimented with tying ligatures (silk threads) around individual blood vessels to stop bleeding. However, Paré's method took longer than cauterising, and the ligatures could carry infection. It was not until antiseptics were developed (300 years later) that they could be used safely.
Key question 5: How did Hunter change surgery and anatomy?  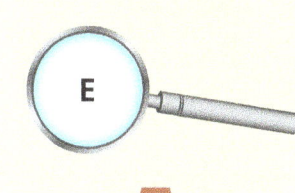 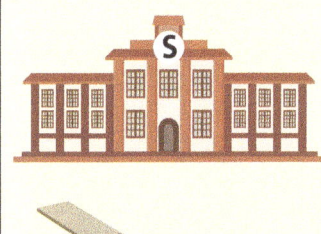 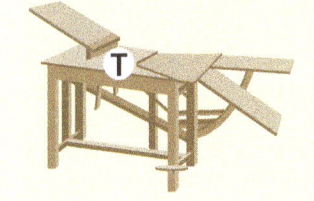	John Hunter became perhaps the **best-known** British surgeon of the eighteenth century. Hunter's fame showed how surgeons were growing in status, and how surgery and anatomy were becoming an important part of medicine. • **Books** – Hunter was surgeon to King George III and this gave him fame and influence. His books on dentistry, venereal disease and the treatment of gunshot wounds were widely read and influenced medical treatments. • **Experimentation** – Hunter encouraged a scientific approach and experimentation. His approach inspired other individuals, such as Edward Jenner (who developed a vaccination against smallpox). • **School** – Hunter set up his own anatomy school and trained hundreds of surgeons. • **Techniques** – Hunter developed new surgical techniques. In one famous case, he successfully treated a man with a tumour on his knee by tying off arteries to restrict the blood flow above the aneurysm (a bulge in a blood vessel). Traditionally, the man would have had his leg amputated.

Core content 2.2: Dealing with disease

Exam specification checklist for this topic

- Methods of treating disease – the use of traditional and new methods
- Quackery
- The Great Plague of London (methods of prevention and treatment)
- The growth of hospitals
- Changes to the training and status of surgeons and physicians

Revision task

Use the flashcards on pages 20–21 to improve your knowledge and understanding of these topics. Test yourself by trying to answer the key questions with the bullet point answers covered up. Make a note of the topics you struggle to remember – you can spend more time on them later in your revision programme.

Key question 1: How did people treat disease during the Plague of 1665?

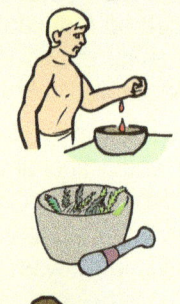

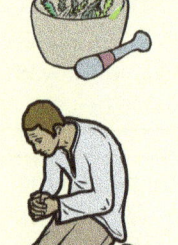

Old methods

- **Bleeding and purging** – These were still the most common treatments. Doctors continued to believe that illnesses were caused when the humours in the patient's body were out of balance.
- **Herbal remedies** – The invention of the printing press led to the widespread publication of 'herbals' (books with ingredients for herbal remedies).
- **Prayer** – Many people still believed that God had sent diseases to punish them for their sins. During the Plague of 1665, the government ordered days of public prayer and fasting so that God would show mercy.
- **Treatments based on superstition** – People continued to wear 'lucky' or 'magical' charms. Superstitious beliefs continued. For example, over 90,000 people visited King Charles II, believing that if he touched them, they would be cured of scrofula (a skin disease known as the 'King's Evil').

New treatments from abroad

European explorers brought back new treatments from around the world. For example:

- **Rhubarb** from Asia was widely used to purge the bowels.
- **Quinine** (extracted from the bark of the cinchona tree from South America) was used to treat fevers. In Britain, it helped many people suffering from malaria.
- **Tobacco** arrived from America and came to be seen as a 'cure-all'. It was recommended for everything from toothache and joint pains to protection from the plague (one schoolboy commented that he was beaten for not smoking enough during the Plague of 1665).

Key question 2: Who were quacks and what treatments did they offer?

- Quacks were **travelling salesmen**. They went from town to town selling pills.
- They had **no medical qualifications**.
- Quackery became very popular in Renaissance Britain. Men like Joshua Ward made a lot of money from selling '**cure-alls**' – pills that they claimed could cure every illness. All Ward's pills did was make people sweat a lot.
- James Morrison also made a lot of money selling his '**Vegetable Pills**'. These contained strong purgatives and caused many deaths due to excessive bowel movements.

Key question 3: How did people try to prevent the spread of the plague?	After the Black Death, plague never completely disappeared. In 1665, an outbreak in London killed around 100,000 people (over a quarter of the population). One reason was that London was so overcrowded and living conditions were dirty and unhygienic. The Mayor of London did his best to stop the plague from spreading. For example: - Victims were shut up in their homes and watchmen stood guard to stop anyone going in or out. - Households were ordered to sweep the street outside their doors. - Pigs, dogs and cats were not allowed inside the city. - Plays and games were banned to stop large crowds gathering. However, these measures did not really work because: - Not enough men could be found to work as watchmen. More than 20 watchmen were murdered by people escaping from houses that had been shut up. - Parliament refused to turn the orders into laws because MPs refused to be shut in their houses. - The government did not see it as its responsibility to stop the spread of the plague. The King and his council left London. They rarely discussed what to do about the plague.
Key question 4: How did hospitals change?	- **Who ran them?** Medieval hospitals were part of monasteries; they closed when Henry VIII shut the monasteries in the 1530s. Some were taken over by town councils or local charities. - **Who did they treat?** Patients were still mainly the poor and the elderly. Rich people preferred to pay for a nurse or a doctor to treat them at home. - **Who treated the patients?** Nursing sisters treated the patients with herbal remedies. They had no medical training. - **How were the patients treated?** Bleeding and purging were common treatments. People with infectious diseases were still not allowed in. - **How many hospitals were there?** The number of hospitals increased in the 1700s. By 1800, most large towns had a hospital. However, only a small percentage of the population was treated or cared for in a hospital. Most people were cared for by a family member or the local wise woman.
Key question 5: How did the training and status of surgeons and physicians change?	During the 1500s and 1600s, most university-trained physicians still followed the Theory of the Four Humours and the work of Galen. However, during the 1700s, things began to change: - Dissections were encouraged and the work of Vesalius and Harvey became accepted. - Medical equipment was improving, for example, better microscopes and the first thermometers. - In a few hospitals, physicians were trained on the wards.

Core content 2.3: Prevention of disease

Exam specification checklist for this topic

- Methods of preventing smallpox before Jenner
- How Jenner developed a vaccination against smallpox
- Why Jenner's work was significant
- Why there was opposition to Jenner's vaccination

Revision task

Use the flashcards on pages 22–23 to improve your knowledge and understanding of these topics. Test yourself by trying to answer the key questions with the bullet point answers covered up. Make a note of the topics you struggle to remember – you can spend more time on them later in your revision programme.

Key question 1: How did Jenner develop a vaccine against smallpox?	• **Observation** – In his work as a doctor in Gloucestershire, Jenner observed that milkmaids who caught cowpox (a mild disease) never got smallpox. • **Experimentation** – Jenner carried out experiments to see if he could use cowpox to prevent smallpox. In one famous experiment, he took cowpox from a mil maid and inserted the matter into a healthy eight-year-old boy called James Phipps. Jenner then inoculated the boy with smallpox, but no disease followed. • **Publishing his findings** – After carrying out over 20 similar experiments, Jenner published his findings, showing other people how to use his new method, which he called vaccination (the Latin word for cow is *vacca*). • **Funding from the government** – The British government gave Jenner £30,000 to develop his work and vaccination became widely used. The number of deaths from smallpox started to fall.
Key question 2: Why was the work of Jenner significant? 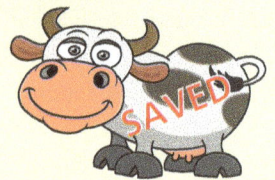	• **Smallpox** – Jenner develop a new method for preventing smallpox. He published his findings in 1798. • **Anti-Vaccine Society** – Jenner's method faced opposition from the Anti-Vaccine Society and it was not until 1853 that the government made vaccination compulsory. • **Vaccinations** – Jenner could not explain why his method worked and, in the short term, vaccinations were not developed to prevent other diseases. However, in the long term (after the discovery of the Germ Theory), other scientists built on Jenner's work and developed vaccines against other diseases. • **Experiments** – Jenner was able to prove his methods worked through experiments. • **Death rates fell** – When the government strictly enforced compulsory vaccinations (after a major smallpox epidemic in 1871) death rates fell dramatically.
Key question 3: Why was there opposition to Jenner's vaccination?	• **Trust** – Jenner could not explain how his vaccination worked and he was not a famous London doctor. • **Fear** – Some physicians reported that Jenner's use of cowpox was having dangerous side effects (causing mutations, such as people sprouting cow hair or developing features resembling a cow). • **Beliefs** – Some people believed that disease was punishment for sin, so the only protection was living a life close to God. Others thought it was forbidden to mix animal matter with human flesh.

Apply: Exam practice

Exam Tip – Question 1: How to evaluate a historical source

How useful is Source A to a historian studying vaccination? (8 marks)

Source A:

Step 1: Use the content of the source
What key features can you see?
- The doctor (possibly Jenner) seems unaware (or perhaps he doesn't care) about the effects the vaccination is having.
- A frightened woman sits in an armchair.
- Small cows leap from shocked patients.
- A boy holds up a bucket of 'Vaccine Pock hot from ye Cow'.

Step 2: Consider the provenance of the source
Identify the following features and explain why each might be useful for the historian.
- **When** the source was produced?
- **Who** produced the source? A cartoonist – not a medical expert but someone who would have been aware of how people were reacting to Jenner's work.
- **Why** did they produce the source? Gilray would have hoped to sell his cartoons – by exaggerating some of the things that people feared about the use of cowpox he might sell more copies.

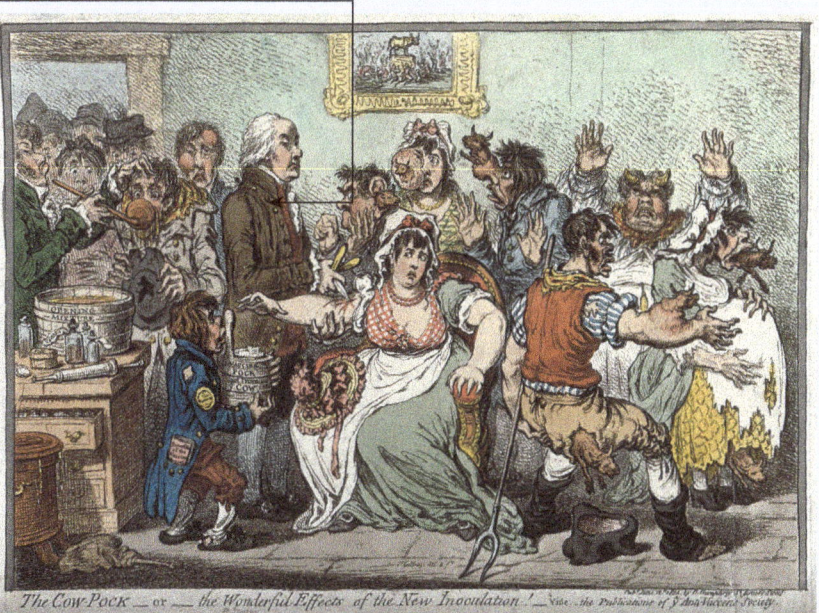

▲ A cartoon drawn by James Gilray in 1802

Step 3: Use your own contextual knowledge to explain why the content and provenance of the source are useful to a historian

Simply describing what you can see in the source will not get you high-level marks. You need to use your knowledge and understanding of the period to place the source in its historical context. Use the planning grid below to help you produce a high-level answer – moving from simple statements to a developed explanation of why the source is useful.

Simple statement	Developed explanation … using your contextual knowledge from the time
The source shows how some people believed that cows would grow out of you if you were vaccinated.	Why did they believe this?
It shows how some people did not trust Jenner's work.	Why was this? It helps us understand that it took time for new ideas to become accepted. When and why did Jenner's ideas become accepted?

Apply: Exam practice

Exam Tip – Question 2: How to explain historical significance

Think before you write using the '4Ds'

Decode – work out the focus of the question

Staying focused on the questions is crucial. If you include information that is not relevant or write about the wrong topic you will waste time and marks. Here's how to 'decode' a question.

What are the command words? The question asks you to 'Explain'. You need to do more than describe; you have to analyse.

Explain the significance of the work of William Harvey in the development of medicine. (8 marks)

What is the content focus? It's about the work of William Harvey but do not simply describe what he did. The focus of this question is on how this work helped medicine develop. This means covering the long-term as well as the short-term importance of his work.

What is the conceptual focus? The concept is **significance**, which means what changed because of Harvey's work? So you need to say briefly what medicine was like before Harvey's discoveries. Then explain how Harvey challenged traditional ideas about physiology. The table you have just produced should help you.

Link Harvey's work with changes that took place in later generations. Aim to **explain** two or three changes that took place.

How many marks are available? There are 8 marks available. This indicates that you should spend about ten minutes on the question and write a couple of paragraphs.

Decide how to organise your answer before you start to write

You do not have the time to tell the story of Harvey's life. The focus is on the **impact** of his work. Decide the main points you want to make and then organise these points into two paragraphs. One possible approach is:

- Paragraph 1: Short-term impact – explain how Harvey challenged Galen's ideas through careful experimentation and dissection.
- Paragraph 2: Long-term impact – explain how others built on Harvey's work and why it was an important breakthrough.

Develop your answer – make sure you explain and support the points you make

Do not simply state that Harvey challenged Galen – explain how and give specific examples.

Do not simply state that Harvey's discoveries were important for many areas of medicine. Explain why they were so important and give examples of how his work is relevant to medicine today.

Demonstrate complex thinking

This earns the top marks in this exam. For example:

- **How fast did change occur?** Do not give the impression that change was instant. Were Harvey's ideas accepted immediately or did the significance of his work take time to be accepted?

Apply: Further exam practice

Use the Exam tips above to plan an answer that explains the significance of Jenner.

Exam Tip – Question 3: How to identify and explain similarities between time periods

Question 3 in the exam asks you to explain similarities between two different time periods.

Look at the two exam questions below. Use your knowledge and understanding of the Middle Ages and Renaissance Britain to answer both questions. The first answer has been started for you.

Explain two ways in which medieval hospitals and hospitals in the 1700s were similar. (8 marks)

This question compares **one area of medicine** (hospitals) in two different time periods.

Focus on **similarities**. Do not go into differences.

When you compare **features** of medicine in different periods you need some key questions to guide you.

Try these questions for hospitals:
1. **Importance**: How many hospitals were there? How many people did they treat? Who did they treat?
2. **Healers**: Who treated patients? Were they trained?
3. **Treatments**: How were patients treated? What methods of treatment were used? How effective were they?

Step 1: Identify the **content focus** of the question

Step 2: Identify the **conceptual focus** of the question

Step 3: Plan
You will have about ten minutes for this 8-mark question in the exam. Aim for two or three well developed paragraphs.

Base each paragraph around a similarity and **make direct comparisons** across the two periods.

DO NOT simply describe one event/period in one paragraph and another event/period in the other!

Explain two ways in which medieval public health and public health in the 1600s were similar. (8 marks)

This question compares **one area of medicine** (public health) in two different time periods.

Focus on **similarities**. Do not go into differences.

When you compare public health features you could focus on the following questions:
1. **Causes**: What caused public health problems?
2. **Development**: How did people respond to public health problems? What role did the government play?
3. **Consequences**: What were the consequences of poor public health? (Think of the Black Death and the Great Plague of London.)

Example answer

Medieval hospitals tended to care for the elderly and the poor. They were small in scale and rarely took in people suffering from infectious diseases. <u>This continued to be the case</u> throughout the Renaissance period, when most hospitals <u>still did not</u> admit people with infectious diseases. Anyone with any money paid for a doctor or nurse to look after them at home. <u>In both periods</u>, the government did not take responsibility for funding and organising hospitals. During the Middle Ages, hospitals were set up by the Church and local charities, while during the Renaissance, they were run by local charities and councils.

There were <u>also similarities in terms of</u> how patients were treated. In hospitals in the Middle Ages ...

Apply: Further exam practice

Explain two ways in which medieval surgery and surgery in the 1700s were similar. (8 marks)

Use the advice on this page to plan how you would approach this question. The PILE memory aid on page 11 might help you.

- Did surgeons face similar problems in both time periods?
- Did surgeons use similar methods in both time periods?

Part 3 The nineteenth century, c1800–1900: A revolution in medicine

Knowledge tests: How much do you know about medicine in the nineteenth century?

Recall challenges

1: Know the key individuals

Task
Match each of the individuals in the box below with the area of medicine that they helped to develop. Note that some individuals influenced more than one area of medicine.

Individual	What areas of medicine did they influence?
Louis Pasteur	**Surgery** – improved anaesthetics – developed chloroform
Robert Koch	**Public health** – campaigned for public health improvements during the first half of the nineteenth century – his reports argued that poverty and poor living conditions caused illness
Paul Ehrlich	**Surgery** – antiseptics – developed carbolic spray and encouraged aseptic surgery
James Simpson	**Public health** – established the link between cholera and dirty water
Joseph Lister	**Public health** – developed a sewer system for London
Edwin Chadwick	**Knowledge of the cause of disease** – linked an individual bacterium to an individual disease (this helped to prove the Germ Theory) and went on to develop a method of staining bacteria to make them easier to study
John Snow	**Treatments and cures** – developed Salvarsan 606 (which honed in on and destroyed the bacteria that caused syphilis). This was the first magic bullet (the first chemical cure for a disease)
Joseph Bazalgette	**Knowledge of the cause of disease and the prevention of illness** – developed the Germ Theory and then went on to produce vaccines for anthrax and rabies

2: The ten-minute quiz

List four reasons why the Germ Theory was important.	List two ways in which Koch played an important role in the battle against infectious disease.	List two vaccines developed by Pasteur.	See pages 28–29 for the answers.	Mark out of 8
List three factors that helped in the hunt for microbes.	List two magic bullets (pills made from chemicals that kill infections inside the body).	List two everyday medical treatments and remedies.		Mark out of 7

List four problems facing surgeons in the early 1800s.	List two anaesthetics developed in the 1800s.	List three reasons why there was opposition to chloroform.	See pages 30–31 for the answers.	Mark out of 9
List three ways in which Lister improved surgery.	List three reasons why there was opposition to Lister's methods.	List three examples of aseptic surgery.		Mark out of 9
List three examples of public health problems in industrial Britain.	List three methods used to prevent the spread of cholera.	List three reasons why there was opposition to public health reforms.	See pages 32–33 for the answers.	Mark out of 9
List three individuals who played an important role in improving public health.	List three other factors that led to public health improvements.	List two Public Health Acts that were introduced.		Mark out of 8

Task

1. Using the table below, cover up the second column and see how much you can remember about medicine in Renaissance Britain. Highlight key points you missed.
2. Now add in information you can remember about the nineteenth century. You can use the **Core content** pages in this chapter close the gaps in your knowledge and understanding.

Theme	Renaissance Britain, c1500–1800	The nineteenth century, c1800–1900
Ideas about the causes of illness	• Religious beliefs still strong • Four humours • Bad air	
Treatments	• Bleeding and purging • Herbal remedies (more herbs from overseas, for example, quinine) • Cures based on superstition	
Surgery and anatomy	• Better knowledge of anatomy (Vesalius) and physiology (Harvey) • No effective antiseptics or anaesthetics • Cauterisation and ligatures to stop bleeding • Improved treatment of gunshot wounds (Paré)	
Public health and methods of prevention	• Some attempts by the Mayor of London to prevent the spread of the plague (1665) • Governments did little to improve public health or stop diseases from spreading • Government funding for Jenner	
Hospitals and healers	• Hospitals still did not deal with infectious diseases • Hospitals set up by charities and local councils • Training began to change and dissection was encouraged • Most medical care was provided by women within the family or the local wise woman	

Core content 3.1: The development of the Germ Theory and its impact on the treatment of disease in Britain

Exam specification checklist for this topic
- The importance of Pasteur's development of the Germ Theory
- The importance of Koch's work microbe hunting
- Paul Ehrlich and the development of magic bullets
- Everyday medical treatments and remedies

Revision task
Use the flashcards on pages 28–29 to improve your knowledge and understanding of these topics. Test yourself by trying to answer the key questions with the bullet point answers covered up. Make a note of the topics you struggle to remember – you can spend more time on them later in your revision programme.

Key question 1: How did Louis Pasteur develop the Germ Theory?

- Louis Pasteur was a French scientist who was asked to investigate why alcoholic drinks, like beer and wine, sometimes went sour. His solution was to heat the drinks briefly to kill off disease-causing bacteria. This became known as **pasteurisation**.
- Pasteur thought that germs from the air were causing the liquids to go sour. He also speculated that germs might be getting into humans and causing disease. Pasteur published his **Germ Theory** in 1861.
- The French government paid for Pasteur to set up a research team to carry out experiments to prove the theory correct. In 1865, Pasteur proved that the disease killing silkworms (used to produce silk) was being spread by germs in the air. This was the first time it was **proved that germs were causing disease in animals**.

Key question 2: How did Robert Koch play an important role in the battle against infectious diseases?

- Robert Koch, a German doctor, built on Pasteur's work. In 1876, Koch's research team made an important breakthrough – identifying the bacterium that was causing anthrax (a disease that affected animals and humans). This was the first time anyone had **identified the specific microbe causing a particular disease**. It was the proof that Pasteur's Germ Theory was correct.
- Koch developed a **method of staining bacteria to make them easier to study**. They could then be photographed using a new, high-quality photographic lens. Koch used this method to identify the tiny bacterium that caused tuberculosis (TB). His methods became widely used and by 1900, scientists had found the bacteria that caused other killer diseases, such as typhoid, pneumonia and plague.

Key question 3: What factors helped in the development of the Germ Theory and the hunt for microbes?

Factor	Examples
Individuals	- Pasteur's genius, determination and experiments - Koch developing a method to stain bacteria
Chance	- Working for the French alcohol industry and silk industry gave Pasteur the opportunity to develop his ideas
Communication	- Koch read Pasteur's research and built on it to identify specific germs that caused a particular disease - Other scientists were able to use Koch's methods to discover bacteria that caused other diseases and vaccines to prevent them
Science and technology	- Pasteur benefited from improved microscopes - Koch used new, high-quality photographic lenses to study bacteria

Key question 4: Why was the development of the Germ Theory so important?	The development of the Germ Theory was a crucial turning point. Not everyone accepted Pasteur's theory straight away. However, over time, it persuaded people that bad air was not the cause of disease. For the first time, doctors understood what really did cause disease and this revolutionised medicine and health care. The Germ Theory made a huge difference. • **Vaccines** – Once specific bacteria had been linked to specific diseases, vaccines were developed to prevent them. • **Acts** – The government introduced Public Health Acts (laws) to improve living conditions (providing fresh water supplies and sewage systems). • **Surgery** became safer – Antiseptics were developed to kill germs during operations and stop infections. Aseptic surgery was developed to make sure that operating theatres were germ free. • **Treatments** – New treatments included chemical drugs (magic bullets) that were developed to destroy the harmful bacteria that caused diseases. In the early twentieth century, antibiotics were developed to kill bacteria in the body.

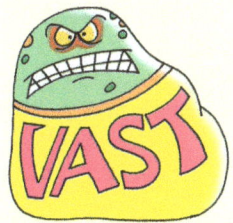

Key question 5: What impact did the Germ Theory have on ways of preventing and treating disease?	Pasteur and Koch's work led to the **development of vaccines to prevent disease**. • Pasteur's research team developed a vaccine against **anthrax**. He tested this successfully in a public experiment and the news spread rapidly around Europe. • Pasteur also developed a vaccine against **rabies**. He tested it successfully on dogs but did not know if it would work on people. The chance to find out came in 1885, when he tested it on a young boy who had been bitten by a rabid dog. Pasteur gave the boy 13 injections over a two-week period. This saved the boy's life. • Other scientists followed Pasteur's work and vaccines were developed against tuberculosis (1906), tetanus (1927), measles (1950s) and polio (1950s). Pasteur and Koch's work also led to the development of the **first chemical cures or 'magic bullets'**. • In 1909, **Paul Ehrlich** (who had been part of Koch's research team) developed the first chemical cure for a disease. This was **Salvarsan 606**, which he called a magic bullet because it homed in on and destroyed the harmful bacterial that caused **syphilis**. Within three years, Salvarsan had cured 10,000 people of syphilis. • In the 1930s, **Gerhard Domagk** developed **Prontosil**, a chemical magic bullet, which could cure **blood poisoning**.

Key question 6: What everyday treatments and remedies existed in the nineteenth century?	• Magic bullets only killed specific bacteria – they could not kill the germs that caused most infections. Despite the work of brilliant individuals such as Pasteur and Koch, improvements in medical knowledge did not lead immediately to new treatments. • Until 1900, most people were still treated at home in traditional ways, using **home remedies**. These treatments still had a lot in common with treatments used in the Middle Ages and Renaissance. • If home remedies did not work, people bought **'patent' medicines**, often known as **'cure-alls'** because they claimed to cure nearly all illnesses. Thomas Holloway became a multi-millionaire selling pills containing ginger, soap and purgatives. Addiction, deaths and illnesses resulting from overdoses were common.

Core content 3.2: A revolution in surgery

Exam specification checklist for this topic
- The development of anaesthetics (including Lister and chloroform)
- The development of antiseptics (including Lister and carbolic acid)
- The development of aseptic surgery and better surgical procedures

Revision task
Use the flashcards on pages 30–31 to improve your knowledge and understanding of these topics. Test yourself by trying to answer the key questions with the bullet point answers covered up. Make a note of the topics you struggle to remember – you can spend more time on them later in your revision programme.

Key question 1: What problems faced surgeons in the early 1800s?

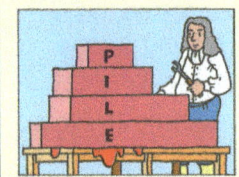

Despite the work of Paré and Hunter, surgeons in the early 1800s still faced the same problems as surgeons in the Middle Ages. The PILE of problems below led to high death rates as patients died from shock of pain, blood loss and infection.
- **Pain** – Surgeons did not have access to effective anaesthetics.
- **Infections** – They had no effective antiseptics to stop infection.
- **Loss of blood** – They did not have fast ways of stopping major bleeding.
- **Environment** – Operating theatres were very unclean and spread germs.

Key question 2: Why was the work of James Simpson significant?

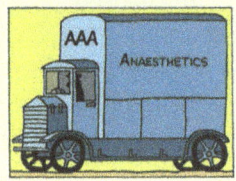

Before Simpson:
- The only way to reduce pain was speed. The patient was held or tied down while the surgeon operated as fast as possible. This led to rushed operations and lots of mistakes.
- In the late 1700s and 1800s, scientists found that some chemicals could work as an anaesthetic and reduce pain. Laughing gas (nitrous oxide) was used but it did not make patients completely unconscious. When it was used in a public demonstration, the patient was in agony. In the 1840s, ether was used as an anaesthetic but it was difficult to inhale, irritated the lungs (causing coughing and sickness) and could catch fire if exposed to a flame.

In the short term:
- Simpson developed a better anaesthetic, called chloroform. This was faster acting and gentler than ether. Simpson wrote articles about his discovery and other surgeons started to use chloroform in their operations, especially after Queen Victoria praised it after she was given chloroform during the birth of her eighth child.
- This meant that surgeons could work more slowly and carefully, without fear that their patients might die from shock. They were also able to carry out more complex operations. However, there was opposition to anaesthetics (see Key question 5) and longer operations meant an increased risk of infection and higher death rates.

In the long term:
- The effectiveness of chloroform encouraged others to search for better anaesthetics. Other chemicals were used which relaxed muscles. Local anaesthetics were developed which numbed pain in one specific area of the body.

Key question 3: Why was the work of Joseph Lister significant?	**Before Lister:** • Before the Germ Theory, no one knew what was causing infection. This led to dangerous practices by surgeons, such as reusing bandages and using unclean equipment. This spread infection and caused high death rates. **In the short term:** • Pasteur's Germ Theory encouraged Lister to look for ways to kill bacteria in the wound. He saw how carbolic acid was used to treat sewage when it was used to fertilise the land (it killed the parasites that could infect cattle feeding on the land). • Lister carried out experiments – applying carbolic acid to stop infection developing in open wounds and soaking bandages in carbolic acid. He found that the wounds healed and did not develop gangrene. • In 1867, Lister published results which clearly showed the value of using carbolic acid during amputations – death rates were reduced from over 45 to 15 per cent. **In the long term:** • Lister went on to use carbolic spray in every stage of an operation. He encouraged surgeons to wash their hands with carbolic spray before the operation, use carbolic spray to kill germs around the operating table and use ligatures soaked in carbolic acid to tie up blood vessels. • There was opposition to Lister's methods but Lister's demonstrations and teaching (he trained students in Edinburgh and then London) helped to overcome it. By 1900, his ideas were widely accepted, and death rates started to fall in surgery.
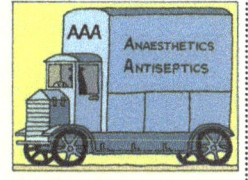	
Key question 4: How did aseptic surgery improve surgery? 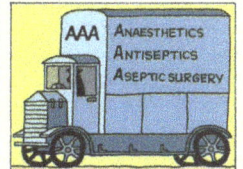	Lister's method, which killed germs on the wound, was called antiseptic surgery. By the 1890s, this had developed into aseptic surgery, which meant removing all germs from the operating theatre. • Operating theatres and hospitals were carefully cleaned. • All surgical instruments were steam-sterilised. • Surgeons wore gowns, face masks and rubber gloves. As a result of antiseptics and aseptic surgery, death rates fell. Also, surgery became more ambitious. For example: • 1880s – first successful operation to remove an appendix • 1890s – first heart operation.

Key question 5: Why did Simpson and Lister face opposition?	Reasons for opposition to Simpson's methods	Reasons for opposition to Lister's methods
	The methods were new and untested. When Hannah Greener died during an operation to remove a toenail, it scared surgeons.	Some surgeons did not achieve the same results as Lister. This was usually because they were less careful.
	Some people thought that pain had been invented by God and it was a good thing to have to endure it during childbirth or an operation.	The new methods caused extra work and slowed down operations.
	Death rates increased. As surgeons carried out longer and more complex operations, it increased the risk of infection.	Surgeons thought carbolic acid was unpleasant – it smelt and cracked the surgeon's skin.

Core content 3.3: Improvements in public health

Exam specification checklist for this topic

- Public health problems in industrial Britain
- Cholera epidemics
- The role of public health reformers (Chadwick)
- Local and national government involvement in public health improvement, including the 1848 and 1875 Public Health Acts

Revision task

Use the flashcards on pages 32–33 to improve your knowledge and understanding of these topics. Test yourself by trying to answer the key questions with the bullet point answers covered up. Make a note of the topics you struggle to remember – you can spend more time on them later in your revision programme.

Key question 1: What public health problems did people face in industrial Britain?

Problem	Causes
Low life expectancy in cities – working class people in Liverpool lived to an average age of 15.	• Overcrowded living conditions • Lack of sewage systems – human waste ended up in the river • Lack of a clean water supply
Cholera epidemics – the epidemic of 1848–49 killed over 50,000 people. There were four major epidemics between 1831 and 1868.	• Drinking unclean water – germs from cesspits infected the water supply • In cities, many people got their drinking water from the river – this was where they dumped their rubbish
The Great Stink of 1858 – this scared Londoners as many people believed that bad air carried disease.	• A very hot summer – a thick layer of sewage lay on the water in the River Thames and the smell of the river became unbearable

Key question 2: What methods were used to prevent the spread of cholera?

Before the Germ Theory, people did not know that germs infected the water supply. Responses to cholera were therefore a familiar mix of common sense and supernatural remedies.

- To protect against bad air: burning barrels of tar, inhaling vinegar, smoking cigars
- Praying to God or wearing lucky charms
- Burning the clothes and bedding of victims
- Quarantine – guards stopped poor people from entering the city

Key question 3: What role did individuals play in encouraging public health reform?

Individual	What did they do?	What impact did they have?
Edwin Chadwick	• Produced reports in the 1840s that linked low life expectancy with poor living conditions. • Argued that people should pay higher taxes to improve sewage systems, remove rubbish from the streets and provide clean water supplies.	• Faced a lot of opposition (especially from taxpayers). • However, after the 1848 cholera epidemics, the government did pass a Public Health Act (see Key question 4).
John Snow	• Produced a book (in 1849) in which he argued that cholera spread through water, not in 'bad air'. • In 1854, produced a report into over 500 deaths from cholera around Broad Street (in London). He linked all the deaths to a water pump on the street (where a nearby cesspool was leaking into the drinking water).	• Snow proved the link between the water and cholera but could not explain why there was a link. (The link was not made until Pasteur published his Germ Theory.) • His work showed the importance of using data to study epidemics and added to the pressure for clean water supplies.

	Octavia Hill	• Campaigned for laws that would force local councils to improve housing. • Bought three London slum houses in 1865 and cleaned them to show landlords how to provide healthy homes. • Went on to buy and improve over 2000 houses.	• Similar schemes were set up in other towns and cities. • In 1875, the government passed the Artisans' Dwelling Act. This gave councils the power to knock down slum housing if it was believed to be unhealthy.

Key question 4: When and why did public health finally improve?

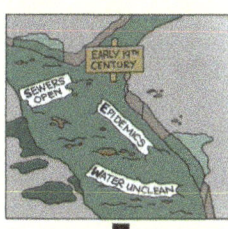

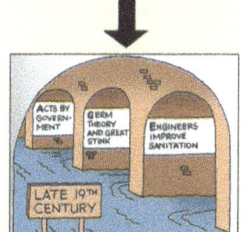

Look at the memory aid, which summarises the main public health changes in the nineteenth century.

In the early 1800s, there were many problems:

Sewers were open and rubbish was thrown into rivers and the streets.

Epidemics such as cholera were very common and killed thousands of people.

Water supplies were unclean – many people got their water from the nearest river or water pump. Some water pumps were very close to cesspits where human waste was dumped.

In the second half of the 1800s, things started to improve:

Acts (laws) were introduced by the government. The Public Health Act in 1848 encouraged change, but it did not force local councils to act. Most local councils did little. However, the 1875 Public Health Act forced local councils to improve sewers, provide fresh water supplies and appoint inspectors to check the new facilities.

Germ Theory and the Great Stink acted as a trigger for action – they changed attitudes and encouraged councils to make improvements.

Engineering improvements were used to build a new sewage system for London. Joseph Bazalgette designed 83 miles of large underground sewers. Pumping stations were built at regular intervals to pump the sewage out of the city.

Exam Tip – Question 4: How to evaluate the key factors

For Question 4 in the exam you will need to think carefully about the language you use to describe the role played by the factors that influence changes in medicine and health care. Aim to choose words that show the examiner that you recognise that some causes/factors are more important than others.

Task

What factors played an essential role in improving public health?

Complete the factors table below by filling in the third column. Decide whether you think the factor was:
- essential (no change would have happened without it)
- important
- minimal (it only had a small impact).

Factors in improving public health	What role did this factor play?	How important was this factor?
Individuals	(See Key question 3)	*Important – they highlighted problems and put pressure on the government to change things*
Chance events	• Cholera epidemics • The Great Stink	
Science and technology	• Germ Theory • Improvements in engineering	
Government	• Public Health Act in 1848 • Public Health Act in 1875	

Apply: Exam practice

Revisiting Question 1: How to evaluate a historical source

Use the Exam tip box on page 23 and the advice below to answer the following exam question.

Study Source A. How useful is Source A to a historian studying surgery in the late nineteenth century?

(8 marks)

Step 1: Use the content of the source

What key features can you see?

- The surgeon is very calm and focused – the operation does not appear to be rushed.
- An assistant is using chloroform on a cloth to anaesthetise the patient.
- Another assistant mops up blood with a sponge.
- Carbolic spray disinfects the area.
- The surgeon and his assistants are not wearing gloves, masks or gowns.

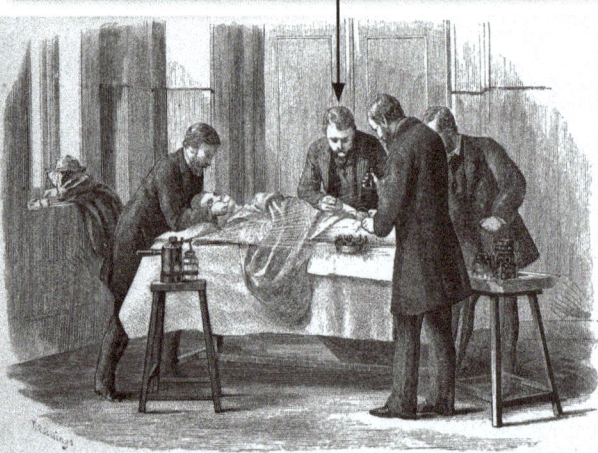

▲ **Source A** This picture shows an operation taking place while a carbolic spray disinfects the area. The picture comes from a textbook for surgeons called *Antiseptic Surgery*, produced by William Watson Cheyne in 1882. Cheyne was an experienced surgeon at King's College Hospital, London (where Lister worked from 1877), and was a keen supporter of Lister's methods.

Step 2: Consider the provenance of the source

Identify the following features and explain why each might be useful for the historian.

- **When** was the source produced? In this case 1882, 15 years after Lister had published his research. At the time, there was some opposition to Lister's methods, but his ideas were starting to be widely used.
- **Who** produced the source? An experienced surgeon from the hospital in London where Lister worked and a supporter of Lister's methods.
- **Why** did they produce the source? The picture was part of a textbook that Cheyne produced to train less experienced surgeons.

Step 3: Use your own contextual knowledge to explain why the content and provenance of the source are useful to a historian

Complete the planning grid below to help you produce a high-level answer – moving from simple statements to a developed explanation of why the source is useful.

Simple statement	Developed explanation … using contextual knowledge from the time
The source shows the use of … during operations.	The fact that Lister's methods are being demonstrated in a textbook to train surgeons shows that by the end of the 1880s his ideas were becoming accepted. This was beacause…
The source also shows the use of … as an anaesthetic.	This had been developed by Simpson. He initially faced some opposition, however, the source shows us that by the 1880s, chloroform was being widely used. The use of antiseptics alongside anaesthetics marked a turning point in surgery because…
However the source indicates that in the 1880s, aseptic surgery had not been fully developed.	There is no evidence of…

Apply: Exam practice

Revisiting Question 2: How to explain historical significance

Remind yourself of the approach you took to planning your answers to the significance question on page 24, then answer the two questions below.

- Explain the significance of the Germ Theory in the development of medicine in Britain. **(8 marks)**
- Explain the significance of the work of Joseph Lister in the development of surgery. **(8 marks)**

Revisiting Question 3: How to identify and explain similarities between time periods

Question 3 in the exam asks you to explain similarities between two different time periods.

Look at the two exam questions below. Use your knowledge and understanding of the nineteenth century and Renaissance Britain to answer both questions.

Explain two ways in which the work of Simpson and Paré were similar. **(8 marks)**		Explain two ways in which public health in the Renaissance and public health in the early 1800s were similar. **(8 marks)**
This question compares **one area of medicine** (surgery) in two different time periods.	Step 1: Identify the **content focus** of the question	This question compares **one area of medicine** (public health) in two different time periods.
Focus on **similarities**. Do not go into differences.	Step 2: Identify the **conceptual focus** of the question	Focus on **similarities**. Do not go into differences.
When you compare the work of individuals in different periods you could focus on the following questions. 1 **Methods:** How did they make their discoveries? Did they use observation and experimentation? Was there an element of chance? 2 **Impact:** Were their ideas quickly adopted? Did they face opposition? Were there any limitations to their work? (In the case of the question above, think of how the work of both individuals led to an increased risk of infection.) 3 **Factors** that helped them: Did similar factors help them develop their ideas? For example, both Paré and Simpson benefited from improvements in science and technology. Explain why.	Step 3: **Plan** You will have about ten minutes for this 8-mark question in the exam. Aim for two or three well developed paragraphs. Base each paragraph around a similarity and **make direct comparisons** across the two periods. DO NOT simply describe one event/period in one paragraph and another event/period in the other!	When you compare public health features you could focus on the following questions: 1 **Causes:** What caused public health problems? In this case, you could focus on the lack of clean water supplies and effective sewage systems. 2 **Development:** How did people respond to public health problems? What role did the government play? 3 **Consequences:** What were the consequences of poor public health? (Think of the Great Plague of London and the cholera epidemics.)

Part 4 Modern medicine, c1900–today

Knowledge tests: How much do you know about modern medicine?

Recall challenges

1: Know the key individuals

Task
Match each of the individuals in the box below with the area of medicine that they helped to develop. Note that some individuals influenced more than one area of medicine.

Individual	What areas of medicine did they influence?
Alexander Fleming	**Public health** campaigners who linked poverty to ill health and influenced the Liberal government (which introduced reforms 1906–14)
Howard Florey and Ernst Chain	**Surgery and treatments** – helped to develop X-rays and researched radium (used to diagnose and treat cancers)
James Watson and Francis Crick	**Surgery** – used plastic surgery to repair facial injuries during the First World War
Harrold Gillies	**Treatment** – discovered that penicillin kills bacteria (1928)
Archie McIndoe	**Public health** – wrote a report (during the Second World War) recommending that the government set up a national health service
Marie Curie	**Treatment** – gained funding from the British and US governments to manufacture penicillin (1930s and 1940s)
Seebohm Rowntree and Charles Booth	**Surgery** – used skin grafts to reconstruct airmen's faces and hands during the Second World War
William Beveridge	**Knowledge of the cause of disease** – discovered DNA in 1953

2: The ten-minute quiz

List three factors that helped Fleming discover penicillin.	List three factors that helped in the development of penicillin into a mass-produced drug.	List three ways in which the pharmaceutical industry improved treatments.	See pages 38–39 for the answers.	Mark out of 9
List two consequences of the discovery of DNA.	List three new problems that have emerged during the last 100 years.	List two traditional remedies used today.		Mark out of 7

36

List three ways in which surgery improved during the First World War.	List two things that helped surgeons deal with the problem of blood loss.	List three examples of how developments in science and technology have improved surgery.	See pages 40–41 for the answers.	Mark out of 8
List two ways in which Marie Curie made a significant contribution.	List four individuals who have helped to improve surgery since 1500.	List three examples of how war has led to improvements in surgery since 1500.		Mark out of 9
List three individuals who produced reports recommending public health improvements.	List three public health reforms introduced by the Liberal government before the First World War.	List three factors that led to the NHS being established in 1948.	See pages 42–43 for the answers.	Mark out of 9
List three reasons why the introduction of the NHS was significant.	List two reasons why there was opposition to the introduction of the NHS.	List three ways in which the NHS has changed since it was introduced.		Mark out of 8

Task

1 Using the table below, cover up the second column and see how much you can remember about medicine in nineteenth-century Britain. Highlight key points you missed.

2 Now add in information you can remember about the twentieth century. You can use the **Core content** pages in this chapter to close the gaps in your knowledge and understanding.

Theme	The nineteenth century, c1800–1900	Modern medicine, c1900–today
Ideas about the causes of illness	Reached a turning point: • The Germ Theory replaced bad air as an explanation for disease • Microbes that cause individual diseases were identified	Another turning point: In the 1950s …
Treatments	More continuity than change: • Everyday treatments remained the same (for example, herbal) • Patent medicines were not effective	Magic bullets (for example, Salvarsan 606 and Prontosil) The key turning point was the development of …
Surgery and anatomy	Revolutionised after 1840: • Pain – anaesthetics (for example, chloroform) • Infection – antiseptics (for example, carbolic acid) • Environment – start of aseptic surgery	Improvements continue: During the First World War … In the Second World War … In recent years …
Methods of prevention	• 1850s – smallpox vaccinations compulsory • 1880s – new vaccinations (for example, anthrax and rabies)	Widespread use of vaccinations: For example, tuberculosis (1906), diphtheria (1913), … and more recently …
Public health	Improvements after 1840: • Public Health Acts (1848 and more significantly 1875) • 1860s – London sewer system	Liberal reforms (1906–14), for example, … A major turning point in 1948 was the establishment of …

Core content 4.1: Modern treatment of disease

Exam specification checklist for this topic

- Penicillin – its discovery by Fleming and its development
- The development of the pharmaceutical industry
- New diseases and treatments, and antibiotic resistance
- Alternative treatments

Revision task

Use the flashcards on pages 38–39 to improve your knowledge and understanding of these topics. Test yourself by trying to answer the key questions with the bullet point answers covered up. Make a note of the topics you struggle to remember – you can spend more time on them later in your revision programme.

Key question 1: How did Alexander Fleming discover penicillin?

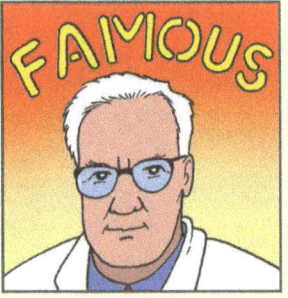

- **War** – provided the motivation for Fleming. During the First World War, he observed many soldiers dying from wounds infected with bacteria (despite antiseptics being used). When he came back from the battlefields, Fleming worked on finding a way to deal with these bacteria.
- **Chance** – provided an opportunity for a key breakthrough in 1928. When he went on holiday, Fleming left a pile of petri dishes containing bacteria on his laboratory bench. On his return, Fleming noticed mould on one of the dishes and that around the mould, the bacteria had disappeared.
- **Individual genius** – Fleming carried out experiments, using microscopes, to observe the impact of the penicillin mould. He discovered that it killed many germs without harming living cells. He used penicillin successfully to treat another scientist's eye infection.
- **Communication** – Fleming stopped his research because penicillin did not seem to work on deeper infections, and it took so long to create enough penicillin to use in his experiments. However, he published his research in a medical journal in 1929. His work was read by Florey and Chain who developed Fleming's idea into an effective medical treatment.

Key question 2: What other factors led to the development of penicillin and antibiotics for everyone?

- **Individuals** – Howard Florey and Ernst Chain were working together at Oxford University in the 1930s. They tested penicillin on mice and discovered that it helped mice recover from infections. In 1941, they tested penicillin on a policeman who had blood poisoning. It worked and the policeman began to recover but then the penicillin ran out and the man died.
- **US government** – Florey and Chain had proved that penicillin worked and that it was not harmful to the patient. The problem was that they needed a lot of funds to mass produce penicillin. Florey travelled to America and persuaded the government to invest in penicillin.
- **War** – The United States government realised the potential of penicillin for treating wounded soldiers in the Second World War. US companies received loans from the American government to buy the expensive equipment needed to produce penicillin on a large scale.
- **Science and technology** – After the war, pharmaceutical companies paid for researchers to discover and trial other antibiotics. Teams of scientists and new technological equipment led to antibiotics being made available for the whole population.
- **British government** – In Britain, after 1948, the government-funded NHS provided antibiotics free of charge. These antibiotics have saved millions of lives.

Key Question 3: How did Fleming become famous?	**F**	**Fleming** – discovers that penicillin mould kills bacteria in 1928
	A	**Antibiotic** – penicillin becomes the first effective antibiotic
	M	**Microscopes** – helped Fleming see that penicillin mould killed many germs
	O	**Other people** – Florey and Chain developed Fleming's idea into a medical treatment
	U	**USA** – funding from the United States paid for the equipment needed to mass produce penicillin
	S	**Soldiers** – Penicillin was widely used to treat soldiers during the Second World War
Key question 4: What role has the pharmaceutical industry played in the development of new treatments?		• Developed the equipment and methods needed to mass produce penicillin.
		• Paid for research to discover and trial new antibiotics.
		• Invested in the development of other treatments. For example, in the 1970s, scientists found that aspirin helped to thin the blood and could help to prevent blood clots. More recent research has shown that it can reduce the risk of a heart attack.
Key question 5: How has our understanding of disease improved in the last 100 years?		• In 1953, Francis Crick and James Watson discovered the structure of human **DNA** and how it passes from parents to children. This was a major breakthrough, showing that many illnesses have genetic causes (for example, diabetes, Parkinson's and many forms of cancer).
		• In the 1990s, the **Human Genome Project** began working out how each part of human DNA affects the body. This has allowed scientists to find ways of treating specific genetic illnesses.
Key question 6: What new diseases and threats have emerged in the last 100 years?		• **Unsafe drugs** – For example, in the late 1950s, **thalidomide** was introduced as a 'safe' sleeping tablet and was given to women to reduce morning sickness during pregnancy. However, the drug had not been fully tested and led to children being born with deformed limbs. The impact led to the more thorough testing of drugs today.
		• **Antibiotic resistance** – For example, **MRSA** is resistant to antibiotics. This shows how overuse of antibiotics has made them less effective.
		• **New diseases** – For example, more than 40 million people have died from **AIDS**-related illnesses. However, in the 1990s, new treatments such as HAART (highly active anti-retroviral therapy) were introduced and these have helped improve survival rates.
Key question 7: What alternative treatments have emerged in the last 100 years?		Some people think that we have become over-reliant on drugs to treat illness and that alternative treatments provide a better solution. For example:
		• **Acupuncture** (which has been used in China for 4000 years) is used to treat disease and as a painkiller during surgery.
		• **Herbal remedies** (many of which have been used in medicine for centuries) are made from plants and animal substances and are available to buy.

Core content 4.2: The impact of war and technology on surgery

Exam specification checklist for this topic

- The development of blood transfusions and X-rays during the First World War
- The development of plastic surgery during the First and Second World Wars
- The development of transplant surgery
- Modern surgical methods, including radiation therapy, transplant and keyhole surgery

Revision task

Use the flashcards on pages 40–41 to improve your knowledge and understanding of these topics. Test yourself by trying to answer the key questions with the bullet point answers covered up. Make a note of the topics you struggle to remember – you can spend more time on them later in your revision programme.

Key question 1: How did the First World War lead to improvements in surgery?

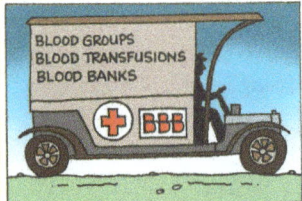

- **X-rays became widely used** in the First World War. Many soldiers had bullets or shrapnel embedded deep in the body and X-rays helped doctors find them quickly before they caused infection. By 1916, all British army hospitals and ambulances were using X-rays.
- **Antiseptics improved** as surgeons in the war began to experiment with new ways of treating infection in wounds. For example, the **Carrel-Dakin method** (named after two doctors) kept a chemical solution flowing through the wound to fight infection.
- **New ways of storing blood developed.** In 1901, Karl Landsteiner had discovered blood groups. This showed why, in the 1800s, some blood transfusions did not work (the blood of some groups cannot be mixed with blood of a different group).

The problem at the start of the war was that when doctors tried to store or transport blood it clotted and could not be used. This was solved by adding **sodium citrate** to prevent the blood from clotting.

Later in the war, scientists discovered how to separate and store the blood cells from plasma and keep them in a **blood bank** for future use.

Key question 2: How did plastic surgery develop in the First and Second World Wars?

In the First World War:

- Plastic surgery improved as surgeons experimented with new ways to repair the damage caused by bullets and shrapnel, particularly to the face and the head.
- **Harrold Gillies** set up a specialist facial injury care unit for wounded soldiers in Kent.
- Surgeons developed new techniques using jaw splints, wiring and metal plates as 'replacement' cheeks.

In the Second World War:

- Plastic surgeons developed new methods to treat burns victims (mainly those who fought in planes or tanks).
- **Archie McIndoe** (a consultant in plastic surgery to the RAF) carried out 4000 operations on burns victims. He used skin grafts to reconstruct airmen's faces and hands.

Key question 3: How did radiation therapy and chemotherapy improve the treatment of cancer?	• Radiation therapy (or radiotherapy) was developed soon after the discovery of X-rays. It uses high energy rays, such as X-rays, to destroy cancer cells. • Since the 1970s, chemotherapy has been used if cancer has developed so far that radiotherapy is not successful. Powerful chemicals are used to attack cancer cells.

Key question 4: How has better science and technology improved modern surgery?	
P = Plastic surgery	• Developed by surgeons in the First and Second World Wars (see Key question 2).
L = Loss of blood	• Tackled by effective **blood transfusions**, which were made possible by to the discovery of **blood groups** and methods of storing blood (**blood banks**) (see Key question 1).
A = Anaesthetics	• Improved by Helmuth Wesse who, in the 1930s, developed anaesthetics that could be injected into the blood stream. Later in the twentieth century, **local anaesthetics** were developed, meaning that operations could take place without the patient being put to sleep.
S = Scanners	• Developed, for example, **X-rays** that made it possible to see inside the body without surgery. Today, CT (computerised tomography) scanners can take thousands of X-ray readings in a second. **MRI** (magnetic resonance imaging) uses magnet and radio waves (rather than X-rays) and can detect cancer cells. Ultrasound scanners can assess the blood flow in veins and arteries.
T = Transplants	• Developed, for example, in 1967, the first **heart** transplant was carried out; **kidney** and **liver** transplants had already been carried out. The early 1980s saw the first bone marrow transplant and the first heart and lung transplant.
I = Infection	• Reduced by improved antiseptic techniques such as the **Carrel-Dakin method** (see Key question 1).
C = Computers	• Helped, for example, **keyhole surgery**, which allows surgeons to work through a tiny hole to carry out complex operations. This is possible because of miniaturisation – all the surgeon's tools are inside an endoscope which is controlled by the surgeon from outside using miniature cameras, fibre-optic cables and computers.
	Also, surgeons can now use robots to carry out some operations. **Nanobots** (tiny specialised robots less than a millimetre long) can perform tasks such as clearing arteries.

Core content 4.3: Modern public health

Exam specification checklist for this topic

- The importance of Booth, Rowntree and the Boer War
- The Liberal social reforms
- The impact of two world wars on public health, poverty and housing
- The Beveridge Report, the welfare state and the creation and development of the National Health Service
- Costs, choices and the issues of health care in the twenty-first century

Revision task

Use the flashcards on pages 42–43 to improve your knowledge and understanding of these topics. Test yourself by trying to answer the key questions with the bullet point answers covered up. Make a note of the topics you struggle to remember – you can spend more time on them later in your revision programme.

Key question 1: What role did the Boer War and public health reformers play in influencing public health in the early twentieth century?

By 1900, life expectancy had only reached 46 for men and 50 for women and the government gave no help to the sick, the unemployed or the elderly. Three events demonstrated the need for change.

- **The Boer War** – When the government tried to raise an army for the Boer War (1899–1902) it found that 38 per cent of recruits were unfit to serve on medical grounds.
- **Rowntree** published a study that showed that more than 25 per cent of the population of York were living in poverty and that this was seriously harming their health.
- **Booth** discovered that 35 per cent of people in the East End of London were living in poverty. He argued that the government should take responsibility for supporting these people and that old-age pensions should be introduced.

Key question 2: What reforms did the Liberals introduce between 1906 and 1914?

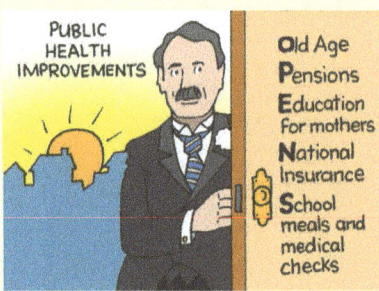

In 1906, a new Liberal government was elected. In their election campaign, the Liberals had promised to tackle poverty and David Lloyd George (the Chancellor) argued that taxes should be raised to pay for the following public health reforms:

- **Old-age pensions** were introduced for people over 70 who did not have enough money to live on.
- Health visitors were employed to **educate new mothers** on how to protect their baby's health.
- The **National Insurance Act** (1911) gave workers medical help if they could not work as a result of illness. The National Insurance scheme required the worker, the employer and the government to pay into a sickness fund. If a worker became too ill to work, they received money and free medical care from the fund. This was a significant step forward, but it only covered people in work (not their families).
- **Free school meals and medical checks** were introduced for school children. Clinics were set up to provide medical treatment for children in school.

Key question 3: What impact did the two world wars have on public health, poverty and housing?	**Improvements in housing:** • During the First World War, the government had promised 'Homes fit for heroes' for the returning soldiers. In 1919, the government introduced a Housing Act – this forced local councils to provide good homes for working people to rent. • In the early 1920s, a quarter of a million new homes were built. In the 1930s, many slum houses were demolished and another 700,000 new houses were built. **The Beveridge Report** – During the Second World War, the government had to provide free health care to keep the country running. It asked William Beveridge to write a report on what should be done to improve people's lives after the war. His main recommendations were for the creation of a **welfare state** that would provide: • **Universal national insurance** to pay benefits (sick pay, old-age pensions, unemployment pay) to everyone, whether they had been workers or not. • **A national health service** that was free to everyone and paid for from taxes. Doctors, nurses and other medical workers would become government employees, instead of charging the sick.
Key question 4: Why was there opposition to the NHS?	• In the 1945 election, the Labour party promised to introduce Beveridge's ideas but it faced opposition from doctors who felt that they would lose their independence and their freedom to treat private patients who paid fees. **Aneurin Bevan** (the new Health Minister) dealt with this opposition by agreeing that doctors could continue to treat patients privately, as well as working for the NHS. • Some people thought that the poor should not be helped. They argued that poor people would grow lazy if they were getting 'something for nothing'.
Key question 5: Why was the introduction of the NHS so significant? 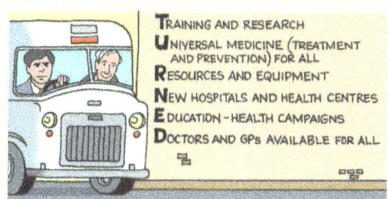	The establishment of the NHS was an important turning point. Britain had **TURNED** an important corner in providing public health facilities. • The NHS spent money on **training** specialist staff and medical research. • It was **universal** – for the first time everyone could get free medical treatment. • The NHS paid for new **resources** and the best medical equipment. • It set up **new hospitals**, health centres and ambulance services. • The NHS ran health **education** campaigns, aiming to prevent illness. For example, there were campaigns warning of the dangers of smoking, an unhealthy diet and lack of exercise. Education campaigns also stressed the importance of vaccinations. • **Doctors**, GPs and nurses now provided free care for everyone.
Key question 6: How has the NHS changed since it was introduced?	• Increasing costs have meant that charges have had to be introduced for prescriptions, dental work and glasses. • The number of hospital beds has been cut. More health care is now provided in the community. • The NHS now focuses on prevention as well as treatment. It runs a comprehensive vaccination programme and has introduced health checks for people over the age of 40. It also educates people about the dangers of smoking, alcohol and obesity.

Apply: Exam practice

Question 4: How to evaluate the key factors

Look at the examples below and notice how you are asked to evaluate how important a **factor** (highlighted in blue) has been in the way that a specific area of medicine (highlighted in orange) has developed from c1000 to the present day.

- Example A: How far has the **government** been the main factor in the development of public health in Britain?
- Example B: Has the role of the **individual** been the main factor in improving the treatment of disease in Britain?
- Example C: How far has **warfare** been the main factor in the development of surgery in Britain?
- Example D: Has **science and technology** been the main factor in understanding the causes of disease in Britain?

Exam Tip 1: Planning your approach to Question 4

Plan your answer using **four paragraphs**. Evaluate the importance of the factor in the question in your first paragraph. Then weigh how important it was compared to two other factors (spend a paragraph on each factor). Finally, come to a conclusion in which you reach a judgement on whether the factor in the question was the main factor.

The example below shows you a good way of planning an answer to **example question A** above (where the focus is on the development of public health). Filling in a quick factors table can help you to ensure that you are exploring a range of time periods. **Use evidence from all four time periods** to support your answer. You do not have to do this in every paragraph but make sure you select your evidence carefully and show off your knowledge of all four periods.

Factors in the development of public health in Britain	The Middle Ages, c1000–1500	Renaissance Britain, c1500–1800	The nineteenth century, c1800–1900	Modern medicine, c1900–today
Government	• Towns employed rakers and made laws but struggled to keep the streets clean	• Attempts by the Lord Mayor of London to stop the spread of the plague (for example, quarantine houses, bans on large gatherings)	• 1848 and 1875 Public Health Acts • Funding for London sewer system • Smallpox vaccination made compulsory	• Liberal government reforms (1906–14) • NHS (Labour government, 1948) • Public health campaigns
Individuals			• Chadwick • Snow • Hill	• Booth • Rowntree • Beveridge • Bevan
War			• Boer War highlights problems (unfit soldiers)	• First World War – 'Homes fit for heroes' • Second World War – government takes over health care

Exam Tip 2: Communicating your knowledge and understanding about causation

Look at the example paragraph below – it argues that individuals played an important role in the development of public health. When arguing the importance of a factor, you cannot simply say that it was important. You have to prove it was. The paragraph below has two important features that will help you move your answer into the higher levels of the mark scheme.

- It is a **substantiated answer** – this means that that the answer is supported by specific examples – look at the sections **highlighted in blue**.
- It is a **developed answer** – look at the sections **highlighted in red** – the answer explains how each individual had an impact, connecting what they did to a specific outcome that improved public health.

Individuals played an important role in the development of public health. For example, John Snow made an important breakthrough when he linked cholera to infected water in the 1850s. His work on the outbreak of cholera around the Broad Street pump in London showed the importance of using data to study epidemics. It also influenced the government, increasing demands for it to provide clean water and an effective sewage system. In the 1800s and early twentieth century, public health campaigners like Chadwick, Hill, Booth and Rowntree helped to change attitudes towards public health. Chadwick's 1842 report highlighted the link between illness and poor living conditions, and his work encouraged the government to introduce a public health act in 1848. Octavia Hill's efforts to improve housing in London helped to persuade the government to pass the 1875 Artisans' Dwelling Act, giving councils the power to knock down slum housing. Individuals such as Beveridge and Bevan also played an important role in setting up the NHS in 1948. After Beveridge had recommended that the government set up a national health service, Bevan played a key role in gaining popular support for the idea and overcoming opposition from doctors.

Exam Tip 3: Writing an effective conclusion

Aim to reach a clear conclusion. Make sure you **directly answer the question**. Did the factor in the question play the **main** role? If so, to what extent? Was it significantly more important than other factors? Evaluate the importance of each factor **using clear criteria**. Think carefully about:

- **The scale of impact** – How important was the role played by the factor in each time period? Was it crucial or essential to the developments that took place? Or did it act as a catalyst (speeding up changes that were already taking place)?
- **The length of time the factor was important** – Did it play an important role across all four time periods? Did its influence grow or diminish over time? Was there a period when it only had a limited influence or played no real role at all?

The Big Picture of medicine and health, c1000–the present day

Task

The table below provides a summary of the key developments in each time period. You can use it to help you revise in the lead up to the exam in the following ways:

1. **Blank page retrieval.** You have reached the end of your revision programme, so see if you can recreate the table on a blank page, from memory. Check your attempt against the table below, and then fill in anything you have forgotten in a different colour on the version you created from memory. Keep your attempt and then try to recreate the table again from memory in a few days' time. Aim to reduce the number of things you forget to include each time you do the activity.

2. **Identify the role played by factors across time.** Use a coding system (for example: B = Beliefs, G = Government, Ch = chance, Co = Communication, W = Warfare, ST = Science and technology) to indicate which factors played the key role in the developments we have highlighted. We have already highlighted where individuals played an important role (their names are in brackets after the discovery/development).

3. **Check you understand the main memory aids.** Can you use the memory aids to explain the key features of the period?

Theme	The Middle Ages, c1000–1500	Renaissance Britain, c1500–1800	The nineteenth century, c1800–1900	Modern medicine, c1900–today
Ideas about the causes of illness	• Four humours (Hippocrates) • Bad air (miasma) • Astrology – movement of the planets • God – a punishment for sins 4 = Four humours B = Bad air A = Astrology G = God	Lots of continuity: • Religious beliefs still strong • Four humours • Bad air	Reached a turning point: • The Germ Theory (Pasteur) replaced bad air as an explanation for disease • Microbes that cause individual diseases were identified (Koch) VAST	Another turning point: • DNA – genetic causes of disease (Watson and Crick)
Treatments	• Prayers and charms • Remedies using herbs, minerals and animal parts • Bleeding and purging to restore the balance of the humours (Galen's Theory of Opposites) • Rest, exercise and diet	Lots of continuity: • Bleeding and purging • Herbal remedies (more herbs from overseas, for example, quinine for malaria) • Cures based on superstition	More continuity than change: • Everyday treatments remained the same (for example, herbal) • Patent medicines were not effective	A revolution in treatments: • Magic bullets (for example, Salvarsan 606 and Prontosil) • The key turning point = the development of antibiotics (for example, penicillin) FAMOUS

Surgery and anatomy	• Doctors did not question Galen's ideas about anatomy • Simple surgery on visible tumours and wounds • Plants such as opium dulled pain but no effective anaesthetics • Wine, vinegar or honey to clean wounds but could not prevent infections • Cauterisation to stop heavy bleeding 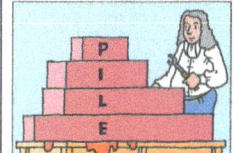	• Better knowledge of anatomy (Vesalius) • Circulation of the blood (Harvey) 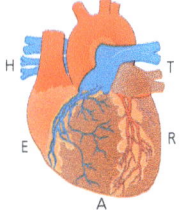 • Cauterisation and ligatures to stop bleeding • Improved treatment of gunshot wounds (Paré) 	Revolutionised after 1840: • Longer and more complex surgery made possible by development of ways to reduce pain and stop infection • Problem of pain solved by the introduction of anaesthetics (for example, ether, chloroform) (Simpson) • Problem of infection solved by the introduction of antiseptics (for example, carbolic acid) (Lister) • The operating environment became safer with the introduction of aseptic surgery (for example, gloves, gowns, masks) 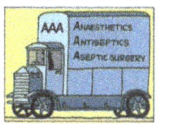	Significant improvements continue: • Further improvements to antiseptics and anaesthetics • Plastic surgery was developed • Blood transfusions became widely used • New equipment and technology transformed surgery – helped with diagnosis (X-rays, scanners, MRIs) and operations (transplant surgery, keyhole surgery)
Public health and methods of prevention	• Kings and governments not expected to improve public health • Epidemic diseases and plagues could not be stopped • Towns employed rakers and made laws but struggled to keep streets clean • Animal and human waste in streets; open sewers; lack of clean water 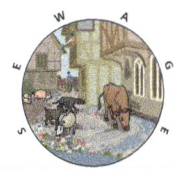	Limited improvement: • Some attempts by the Mayor of London to prevent the spread of the plague (1665) • Governments did little to improve public health or stop diseases from spreading • Vaccine for smallpox (Jenner) but there was opposition to his methods and vaccinations were not made compulsory 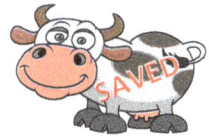	Improvements after 1840: • Public Health Acts in 1848 and more significantly 1875 – government forced councils to take responsibility for sewers and water supply • 1860s – London sewer system (Bazalgette) • 1850s – smallpox vaccinations compulsory • 1850s – cholera linked to dirty water (Snow) • 1880s – new vaccinations 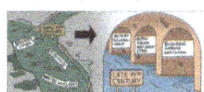	The establishment of the welfare state: • Liberal reforms (1906–14) introduced Old Age Pensions and National Insurance • A major turning point in 1948 with the establishment of the NHS 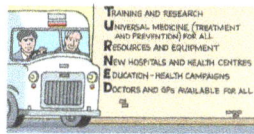 • Widespread use of vaccinations, for example, tetanus (1927), measles (1950s) and Covid (2020)

GLOSSARY

> **Revision Tip**
>
> 1. Look at the nine words highlighted in **BLUE** in the glossary. Link each word to one of the individuals in the bingo card below. Make sure you can explain the link.
>
> | Pasteur | Lister | Simpson |
> |---------|--------|---------|
> | Vesalius | Paré | Jenner |
> | Fleming | Beveridge | Harvey |
>
> 2. Look at the 12 words highlighted in **RED**. Place each word in one of the time periods below:
>
> | The Middle Ages, c1000–1500 | Renaissance Britain, c1500–1800 | The nineteenth century, c1800–1900 | Modern medicine, c1900–today |
> |---|---|---|---|

alternative treatments a way of treating an illness that is not based on mainstream, scientific medicine

anaesthetic a drug or drugs given to produce unconsciousness before and during surgery

anatomy the science of understanding the structure and make-up of the body

antibiotics a group of drugs used to treat infections caused by bacteria, e.g. penicillin

antiseptics chemicals used to destroy bacteria and prevent infection

aseptic surgery the performance of an operation under completely sterile conditions

Black Death a phrase used to describe bubonic plague

carbolic spray used during surgical operations to kill germs in the air around the operating table

cauterise using a hot iron to burn body tissue. This seals a wound and stops bleeding

cholera an infection that causes severe watery diarrhoea (it often results from drinking dirty water)

chloroform a liquid whose vapour acts as an anaesthetic and produces unconsciousness

'cure-all' a medicine usually sold for a profit and often made from a mix of ingredients that had no medical benefits

DNA Deoxyribonucleic acid, the molecule that genes are made of

Germ Theory the theory that germs cause disease, often by infection through the air

keyhole surgery surgical operation performed through a very small incision, using special instruments and an endoscope

ligature a thread used to tie a blood vessel during an operation

'magic bullets' pills made from chemicals that kill particular infections inside the body

NHS a national health service that is free to everyone and paid for from taxes

penicillin the first antibiotic drug, produced from the mould penicillium, used to treat infections

pharmaceutical industry large businesses that mass produce drugs for medicine and health care

physician a doctor of medicine who trained at university

plague a serious infectious disease (bubonic plague was spread to humans by fleas from rats and mice, pneumonic plague was spread by people coughing)

Public Health Acts laws passed to try to improve public health

quack a person who falsely claims to have medical ability or qualifications

radiation therapy or **radiotherapy** treatment of a disease, such as cancer, by the use of X-rays or similar forms of radiation

transfusion the use of blood given by one person to another when a patient has suffered severe blood loss

transplant surgery the implanting of tissue or organs from one part of the body to another, or from a donor to a patient

vaccination the injection into the body of killed or weakened organisms to give the body resistance against disease

Welfare State a system by which a government takes responsibility for the health and well-being of the population

X-ray a photographic or digital image of inside the body